NO MORE WHAT IFS

NO MORE WHAT IFS

How to Master Fear, Follow Your Purpose, and Live Regret-Free

VONLESHIA DAVIDSON

Vonleshia Davidson

NO MORE WHAT IFS

How to Master Fear, Follow Your Purpose, and Live Regret-Free

VONLESHIA DAVIDSON

Vonleshia Davidson

CONTENTS

Copyright	1
Dedication	2
Introduction	4
My Journey: From Fear and Regret to Purpose	8
PART 1: CONFRONTING FEAR AND REGRET (DAYS 1-10)	**13**
Day 1: Identify Your "What Ifs"	14
Day 2: The Root of Fear and Regret	25
Day 3: Changing Your Narrative	37
Day 4: The Courage to Act	55
Day 5: Facing Your Fears	67
Day 6: Letting Go of Regret	78
Day 7: Gratitude Journal	90
Day 8: Self-Talk Audit	102
Day 9: Mindfulness Meditation	114
Day 10: Goal Setting	128

PART 2: EMBRACING YOUR PURPOSE (DAYS 11-20) — 143

Day 11: Discovering Your "Why" — 144

Day 12: Passion Meets Purpose — 156

Day 13: Clarifying Your Vision — 168

Day 14: Crafting Your Purpose Statement — 181

Day 15: Power Poses — 193

Day 16: Review and Refine Purpose Statement — 204

Day 17: Continue Self-Talk Audit/Reframing — 217

Day 18: Mindfulness Meditation/Gratitude Journal — 230

Day 19: Small Wins Celebration — 242

Day 20: Vision Board Completion — 254

PART 3: LIVING A REGRET-FREE LIFE (DAYS 21-30) — 267

Day 21: Integrate Daily Practices — 268

Day 22: Embrace Imperfection — 281

Day 23: Celebrate Your Strengths — 292

Day 24: Cultivate Gratitude — 304

Day 25: Practice Self-Compassion — 317

Day 26: Connect with Others — 330

Day 27: Learn and Grow — 343

Day 28: Embrace Change — 357

Day 29: Trust Your Intuition — 368

Day 30: Live with Intention 380

Conclusion 392

Copyright

Copyright © Vonleshia Davidson 2024
All rights reserved. No part of this book may be reproduced or transmitted in any form or by any means, electronic or mechanical, including photocopying, recording, or by any information storage and retrieval system, without permission in writing from the publisher, except in the case of brief quotations embodied in critical articles or reviews.

Dedication

To my rock, my fortress, my beloved Tim Senior, you are not just a dream that came true, but the dream I hadn't dared to dream. Your unwavering support is the wind beneath my wings, and for that, I am forever indebted. I love you Timber. To my heartbeats, my little wonders, my children - you are the most compelling proof that miracles happen every day. Each sunrise, you teach me the art of becoming a better version of myself. Your smiles are the symphony that orchestrates my life. Mommy loves you, infinitely. To my tribe, my safe haven, my family and friends - you are the cheerleaders of my life saga. Your faith in me is the melody that tunes my resilience. The strength of your support is my secret superpower, the one I wear on tougher days. To my beacon in the storm, my Lighthouse Church family - you are my timely divine intervention. Your presence in my life has painted my gray skies with the hues of hope, love, and faith. My journey is forever enriched, my life forever changed. To the stars in my night sky, my dear Mommy and Daddy W - your absence is a reminder of the precious moments we shared, now transformed into beautiful memories. I carry your love in my heart, your wisdom in my soul. Rest in peace, knowing your little girl misses you every day. To everyone who's touched my life, thank you. This journey, this book, this life - is a testament to you all.

Introduction

Have you ever lain awake at night, your mind racing with a relentless stream of "what ifs"?

What if I had taken that job offer? What if no one buys it? What if I had pursued my dream instead of playing it safe? What if I had moved away all those years ago? What if this, and what if that.

These questions, while seemingly harmless, can become a mental prison. They feed our fears, amplify our regrets, and paralyze us from taking action. We get stuck in a cycle of endless speculation, second-guessing our choices, and dwelling on missed opportunities.

But what if I told you that there's a way to break free from this trap? What if you could silence those nagging doubts, conquer your fears, and finally start living a life of purpose, passion, and no regrets?

That's exactly what this book is all about.

THE "WHAT IF" TRAP: A UNIVERSAL STRUGGLE

The "what if" trap is not a sign of weakness; it's a universal human experience. We all have dreams we haven't chased, chances we didn't take, and words we wish we had said. But when these "what ifs" start to consume our thoughts, they become a toxic force that holds us back from our full potential.

Fear is often at the root of our "what ifs." We fear failure, rejection, the unknown, and even success itself. These fears can manifest as self-doubt, procrastination, and a reluctance to step outside our comfort zones. Regret, on the other hand, is the haunting feeling that we've made the wrong choices, missed out on something important, or let ourselves down.

Together, fear and regret create a powerful duo that keeps us trapped in a cycle of inaction and dissatisfaction. We become prisoners of our own minds, unable to move forward and embrace the life we truly desire.

YOUR 30-DAY JOURNEY TO FREEDOM

The good news is that you don't have to stay stuck in the "what if" trap. You have the power to rewrite your story, overcome your fears, and create a life that you'll look back on with pride and satisfaction.

"No More What Ifs" is your 30-day guide to making that happen. This book isn't about vague theories or empty promises; it's a practical, step-by-step roadmap for transforming your mindset, embracing your purpose, and taking decisive action.

Over the next 30 days, you'll embark on a journey of self-discovery, learning powerful strategies to:

- **Identify and confront your fears:** We'll delve deep into the root of your "what ifs" and equip you with tools to face them head-on.
- **Release the grip of regret:** You'll learn to forgive yourself for past mistakes, make peace with missed opportunities, and focus on creating a brighter future.
- **Uncover your passions and purpose:** We'll guide you through exercises to discover what truly lights you up and how you can make a meaningful impact on the world.
- **Cultivate unwavering self-belief:** You'll develop the confidence to take risks, pursue your dreams, and silence the inner critic that holds you back.
- **Make empowered choices:** You'll learn to make decisions that align with your values and goals, so you can look back on your life with no regrets.

THE POWER OF PURPOSEFUL LIVING

Living with purpose is not just about achieving external goals; it's about aligning your actions with your values, passions, and deepest desires. It's about waking up each day with a sense of excitement and knowing that you're making a difference in the world.

When you live with purpose, fear and regret lose their power. You become less concerned with what others think and more focused on what truly matters to you. You gain the courage to take risks, the resilience to overcome setbacks, and the unwavering belief that you are capable of achieving great things.

This book is not a magic pill; it requires commitment, effort, and a willingness to step outside your comfort zone. But if you're ready to break free from the "what if" trap, embrace your purpose, and create a life that you'll love, then this 30-day journey is for you.

Let's get started.

My Journey: From Fear and Regret to Purpose

Hey, Friend. Pull up a seat and lean in close because I've got a story to share with you—*my* story. It's full of unexpected twists, heartbreaks that almost took me out, and victories I didn't see coming. There were fears that kept me up at night and regrets that tried to steal my joy. But let me tell you this—it's also a story of discovering purpose, rising from the ashes, and stepping boldly into a life where "what if" is no longer a question. It's a journey of choosing faith over fear and claiming the promise that's been waiting all along.

Growing up wasn't a walk in the park. I saw the kind of heartbreak most kids only hear about—drug addiction and domestic violence weren't just stories; they were realities unfolding in my own home. By the time I was nine, I was taken from my birth mother and placed into foster care. God had other plans, though, because soon enough, my aunt stepped in and adopted me, raising me as her own. I call her Suga-Momma — that's my girl right there. She, along with my other aunt, stepped up in ways my mother couldn't. They poured into

This book is not a magic pill; it requires commitment, effort, and a willingness to step outside your comfort zone. But if you're ready to break free from the "what if" trap, embrace your purpose, and create a life that you'll love, then this 30-day journey is for you.

Let's get started.

My Journey: From Fear and Regret to Purpose

Hey, Friend. Pull up a seat and lean in close because I've got a story to share with you—*my* story. It's full of unexpected twists, heartbreaks that almost took me out, and victories I didn't see coming. There were fears that kept me up at night and regrets that tried to steal my joy. But let me tell you this—it's also a story of discovering purpose, rising from the ashes, and stepping boldly into a life where "what if" is no longer a question. It's a journey of choosing faith over fear and claiming the promise that's been waiting all along.

Growing up wasn't a walk in the park. I saw the kind of heartbreak most kids only hear about—drug addiction and domestic violence weren't just stories; they were realities unfolding in my own home. By the time I was nine, I was taken from my birth mother and placed into foster care. God had other plans, though, because soon enough, my aunt stepped in and adopted me, raising me as her own. I call her Suga-Momma — that's my girl right there. She, along with my other aunt, stepped up in ways my mother couldn't. They poured into me, tried to shield me from life's storms, and loved me through it all.

But even with all that love wrapped around me, fear still had a seat at the table. It whispered in my ear, planting seeds of doubt and making me question my worth. "Are you even good enough?" it sneered. "Nobody will ever want you." Fear had me stuck, paralyzed by the thought of failure, rejection, and the unknown. It made me play small, dim my light, and doubt every step I took.

But oh, baby, you know how God works, don't you? He's in the business of taking shattered pieces and rewriting stories. He didn't leave me there, stuck in my own doubts. No, He picked up the pen and started crafting a new chapter, one where fear didn't get the final word.

As I journeyed through life, I piled up on my fair share of regrets. I made mistakes in relationships, questioned my choices in both my personal and business life, and even experienced the heartbreak of sacrificing myself for love only to end up feeling lost and unfulfilled.

One chapter in my story that took me to the brink was when my husband and I decided to try an open marriage. Yes, you read that right. We were young, wild, and thought we had it all figured out. Now, don't rush to judge me. We were chasing this idea of freedom and exploration, thinking it would somehow fill the gaps and bring us closer. But sometimes, the pursuit of what feels like freedom only leads to deeper chains.

What we thought would be an exciting journey turned out to be a path filled with more regret and heartache than we anticipated. I realized pretty quickly that I didn't have the heart for that kind of wild life. It wasn't just that it wasn't for us - it left us with a sense of shame and a few scars we hadn't expected. We learned some hard lessons about boundaries and the true cost of stepping outside them. Ultimately, it made us face the fact that not every kind of freedom is worth chasing.

Yet, it was within that melting pot of pain and regret that I discovered a strength I didn't know was in me. It took some deep soul-searching and raw self-reflection to get there, but I came to see that even the most painful experiences had given me something invaluable—a deeper understanding of what it means to be human. I learned to face my fears head-on, challenge the doubts that tried to hold me back, and start making choices that genuinely aligned with my values. It was in those moments of struggle that I began to reclaim my sense of self and redefine what I truly wanted out of life.

As I embarked on my own healing journey, I found solace and guidance in my faith. I began to rely on Jesus Christ as my source of strength, wisdom, and direction. I started consulting Him in every decision, both in my personal life and in my business. This shift in perspective transformed my entire life.

With a newfound sense of purpose and direction, we rebuilt our marriage on a foundation of love, forgiveness, and a renewed commitment to each other. We put in the work to create a beautiful partnership—one that is stronger and more fulfilling than ever before. The lessons from our past became stepping

stones toward a deeper, more authentic connection. Today, we're not just in love; we're closer than ever, having turned our struggles into the very things that made our bond unbreakable.

Alongside healing my marriage, I discovered a burning

passion for helping others overcome their own fears and regrets. I wanted to empower people to pursue their passions and achieve their personal development goals. Drawing upon my life experiences and my bachelor's degree in psychology, I became a certified life and mindset coach. Now, I'm also finishing up my MBA, adding another layer of expertise to support and guide others on their journey to growth and transformation.

I've been able to build my own six figure business and had the privilege of speaking at events around the world, hosting panels on business, mindset and success, and working with over 5,000 women to start their e-commerce businesses and build thriving careers. It's been an incredible journey of empowerment and transformation, both for myself and for those I've had the honor of coaching.

I share my story not to boast, but to show that I genuinely understand the struggles you might be facing. I know what it's like to feel trapped by fear and regret, to question your worth, and to wonder if you'll ever find your path. But I also know, from experience, that transformation is possible. You're looking at a college dropout who went back to school, married with two kids, and will soon have an MBA. Sometimes, I still can't believe it myself. But here's what I've learned: there is a way forward, and it's not just for the lucky or the fearless—it's for anyone willing to face their doubts and fight for a better future.

That's why I wrote this book. It's a culmination of everything I've learned through my own experiences, my education, and my work with countless others. It's a 30-day guide designed to help you break free from the "what if" trap, overcome your fears, discover your purpose, and start living a life that's authentically yours.

This book isn't about becoming someone you're not; it's about embracing your true self, with all your flaws and imperfections. It's about recognizing your inherent worth, unleashing your unique gifts, and using them to make a positive impact on the world.

If you're ready to let go of the past, conquer your fears, and step into a future filled with purpose and possibility, then I invite you to join me on this journey. Together, we'll navigate the ups and downs, celebrate the victories, and learn from the challenges.

And remember, this isn't just a 30-day challenge; it's a lifelong commitment to personal growth, self-discovery, and purposeful living. So, let's dive in, my friend. Your new chapter awaits.

Part 1: Confronting Fear and Regret (Days 1-10)

Day 1: Identify Your "What Ifs"

Welcome to the first day of your journey to "No More What Ifs!" Today, we're going to shine a light on those nagging doubts and lingering regrets that have been holding you back. It's time to confront the "what ifs" head-on and take the first step towards a more empowered and purposeful life.

THE WHISPERS OF DOUBT

Think back to the last time you found yourself caught in a spiral of "what ifs." Maybe it was a job opportunity you passed up, a relationship you didn't pursue, or a dream you never chased. Perhaps you're haunted by past mistakes or missed opportunities, wondering how things could have been different.

These "what ifs" can be like whispers in the back of your mind, casting doubt on your choices and undermining your confidence. They can make you question your abilities, second-guess your decisions, and even paralyze you from taking action.

Part 1: Confronting Fear and Regret (Days 1-10)

Day 1: Identify Your "What Ifs"

Welcome to the first day of your journey to "No More What Ifs!" Today, we're going to shine a light on those nagging doubts and lingering regrets that have been holding you back. It's time to confront the "what ifs" head-on and take the first step towards a more empowered and purposeful life.

THE WHISPERS OF DOUBT

Think back to the last time you found yourself caught in a spiral of "what ifs." Maybe it was a job opportunity you passed up, a relationship you didn't pursue, or a dream you never chased. Perhaps you're haunted by past mistakes or missed opportunities, wondering how things could have been different.

These "what ifs" can be like whispers in the back of your mind, casting doubt on your choices and undermining your confidence. They can make you question your abilities, second-guess your decisions, and even paralyze you from taking action.

But here's the thing: "what ifs" are not facts; they're simply stories we tell ourselves. They're often rooted in fear – fear of failure, rejection, the unknown, or even success itself. And when we give these fears too much power, they can become self-fulfilling prophecies, preventing us from reaching our full potential.

THE "WHAT IF" INVENTORY

The first step to overcoming your "what ifs" is to identify them. It's time to bring those whispers out of the shadows and into the light. Grab a pen and paper, find a quiet space, and let's start uncovering what's been holding you back.

I want you to create a "What If" inventory. Don't hold back. Be honest with yourself about the doubts, regrets, and anxieties that have been swirling around in your mind. Write down everything that comes to mind, no matter how big or small.

Here are some prompts to get you started:

- ***What if I had taken that risk?***
- ***What if I had spoken my truth?***
- ***What if I had pursued my passion?***
- ***What if I had forgiven myself?***
- ***What if I had believed in myself more?***

As you write, notice any patterns or themes that emerge. Are your "what ifs" mainly focused on your career, relationships, personal growth, or something else? This will help you gain deeper insights into the areas of your life where fear and regret have the strongest hold.

Remember, this is not an exercise in self-blame or shame. It's about gaining awareness and understanding so that you can start to move forward. Be kind to yourself as you explore these
thoughts and feelings. It's important to give yourself grace, and don't judge yourself while doing this.

This inventory is your starting point. By identifying your "what ifs," you're taking the first courageous step towards overcoming them. In the coming days, we'll delve deeper into the root causes of your fears and regrets, develop strategies for reframing negative thoughts, and start taking action towards a life of "no more what ifs."

Are you ready to take that step? Let's be honest – we've all fallen prey to the seductive whispers of "what if." Those two little words have an uncanny ability to hijack our thoughts, leaving us trapped in a maze of anxieties, missed opportunities, and crippling self-doubt.

WHAT IFS: THE SHAPE-SHIFTERS OF OUR MINDS

"What ifs" are sneaky little pain in the butt. They can disguise themselves as harmless thoughts, but underneath, they often harbor deep-seated fears and insecurities. They come in various forms, each with its own unique way of undermining our happiness and hindering our progress.

- **The Anxiety-Inducing What Ifs:** These "what ifs" are

like alarm bells that never stop ringing. They focus on potential negative outcomes, painting worst-case scenarios in vivid detail. *What if I fail this exam? What if I get laid off? What if I make a fool of myself? What if I get hurt?* These thoughts trigger anxiety, stress, and a sense of impending doom.

- **The Regret-Fueled What Ifs:** These "what ifs" dredge up the past, reminding us of missed opportunities and paths not taken. *What if I had pursued that dream job? What if I had said "yes" to that date? What if I had invested in that stock?* These thoughts can lead to feelings of regret, guilt, and a lingering sense of "what could have been."

- **The Self-Doubt-Inducing What Ifs:** These "what ifs" chip away at our confidence, questioning our abilities and worthiness. *What if I'm not good enough? What if I don't deserve success? What if they don't like me?* These thoughts breed insecurity, self-doubt, and a reluctance to take risks.

THE VICIOUS CYCLE OF "WHAT IFS"

The danger of "what ifs" is that they perpetuate a vicious cycle. When we dwell on negative possibilities, we create a self-fulfilling prophecy. Our anxieties and doubts can sabotage our efforts, leading to the very outcomes we fear.

This cycle can manifest in various ways:

- **Procrastination:** We put off taking action because we're afraid of failing or making the wrong decision.

- **Missed opportunities:** We hesitate to seize chances because we're worried about the potential consequences.
- **Imposter syndrome:** We doubt our abilities and feel like we don't deserve our successes.
- **Anxiety and depression:** The constant barrage of negative thoughts can lead to chronic stress and mental health issues.
- **Relationship problems:** Our fears and insecurities can create tension and distance in our relationships.

STUCK IN THE PAST OR FEARING THE FUTURE

The "what if" trap is a thief of joy that robs us of the present moment. When we're consumed by anxieties about the future or regrets about the past, we miss out on the beauty and opportunities that surround us right now.

We become prisoners of our own minds, unable to fully engage in our lives or appreciate the present moment. We lose sight of our goals, our passions, and our purpose. We become stuck, unable to move forward and create the life we truly desire.

BREAKING FREE: THE FIRST STEP

The first step to breaking free from the "what if" trap is awareness. It's about recognizing the negative patterns of thought that hold you back and understanding how they manifest in your life. It's about identifying the specific fears and regrets that fuel your "what ifs."

Once you have this awareness, you can start to challenge these thoughts and replace them with more positive and empowering
ones. You can learn to focus on the present moment, cultivate gratitude for what you have, and take action towards your goals, even in the face of fear.

The "What If" Inventory exercise you'll do today is designed to help you gain this awareness. It's a powerful tool for identifying your most common "what ifs" and understanding the underlying emotions that drive them. With this knowledge, you'll be equipped to start breaking free from the "what if" trap and create a life that is intentional, purposeful, and regret-free.

RECOGNIZING YOUR PATTERNS

Now that you've started identifying your "what ifs," let's dive deeper. It's time to play detective and uncover the patterns hiding beneath the surface of those nagging questions.

Think of your "what ifs" as clues. Each one offers a glimpse into your fears, regrets, and unmet desires. By analyzing these clues, you can gain valuable insights into the underlying emotions that are driving your thoughts and behaviors.

SPOTTING THE THEMES

Grab your "What If" Inventory (the one you created on Day 1) and take a closer look. Are there any common themes emerging?

Perhaps your "what ifs" revolve around your career:

- "What if I had pursued a different career path?"
- "What if I had asked for that promotion?"
- "What if I start my own business and fail?"

Or maybe your worries center around relationships:

- "What if I had told them how I really felt?"
- "What if I had stayed in that relationship?"
- "What if I never find love?"

Your "what ifs" might also focus on personal growth and self-improvement:

- "What if I had taken that class/workshop/trip?"
- "What if I had invested more time in my hobbies?"
- "What if I never reach my full potential?"

Identifying these themes is like shining a spotlight on the areas of your life where fear and regret are holding you back. It's a crucial step towards understanding the root causes of your "what ifs" and finding ways to overcome them.

UNCOVERING THE EMOTIONS

Once you've identified the themes, it's time to dig even deeper. What emotions are fueling these "what ifs"? Are you feeling fear, sadness, anger, guilt, shame, or a combination of these?

Fear is a common culprit. Fear of failure, fear of rejection, fear of the unknown – these emotions can drive us to play it safe, avoid taking risks, and settle for less than we deserve. But here's the thing: fear is not the enemy. It's a natural human emotion that can serve as a powerful motivator when harnessed correctly. By understanding your fears, you can learn to face them head-on and use them as a catalyst for growth.

Regret is another powerful emotion that can fuel our "what ifs." Regret is that nagging feeling that we've made the wrong choices, missed out on something important, or let ourselves down. While regret can be painful, it can also be a valuable teacher. By examining our regrets, we can gain insights into our values, priorities, and what truly matters to us.

THE POWER OF AWARENESS

Recognizing the patterns and emotions behind your "what ifs" is incredibly empowering. It gives you a deeper understanding of yourself and why you think and act the way you do. It allows you to take ownership of your thoughts and feelings, rather than being controlled by them.

Once you become aware of these patterns, you can start to challenge them. You can question the validity of your fears, reframe your regrets as learning opportunities, and make conscious choices that align with your true desires and values.

Remember, this is a process. It takes time, patience, and self-compassion. There will be setbacks and moments of doubt. But by staying committed to self-discovery and growth, you can break free from the "what if" trap and create a life that is authentically yours.

So, take a deep breath, grab your journal, and start exploring those patterns. Uncover the emotions that are fueling your "what ifs" and embrace the opportunity for transformation. This is your journey to a life of no more "what ifs," and it all begins with understanding yourself a little bit better.

EXERCISE: "WHAT IF" INVENTORY

Grab a pen and paper, friend. It's time to shine a light on those nagging "what ifs" that have been lurking in the shadows of your mind. This exercise is your first step towards liberation, a chance to uncover the hidden fears and regrets that may be holding you back from living your fullest life.

Remember, this isn't about judgment or self-criticism. It's about self-awareness and understanding. Think of it as a detective mission to gather clues about your inner landscape, so you can better navigate your path toward a life of purpose and "no more what ifs."

Here's how it works:

1. **Create a "What If" List:** Start by brainstorming a list of your most common "what if" questions. Don't hold back – be honest and specific. Write down anything that comes to mind, no matter how big or small, silly or serious. Here are a few prompts to get you started:
    - **Career:** "What if I had pursued my passion instead of taking the safe route?" "What if I had spoken up in that meeting?"
    - **Relationships:** "What if I had told that person how I truly felt?" "What if I had ended that toxic relationship sooner?"
    - **Personal Growth:** "What if I had taken that

class/workshop/trip?" "What if I had invested more time in my hobbies?"
- **Health & Wellness:** "What if I had taken better care of my health?" "What if I had started that exercise routine?"

2. **Categorize Your "What Ifs":** Once you have a comprehensive list, start grouping your "what ifs" into categories. This will help you identify patterns and common themes. For example, you might have a category for career-related "what ifs," relationship-related "what ifs," and so on.

3. **Identify the Underlying Emotions:** For each "what if," ask yourself: "What emotion am I feeling when I think about this?" Is it fear of failure? Fear of rejection? Regret for missed opportunities? Identifying these emotions will help you understand the root causes of your "what ifs."

4. **Challenge Your "What Ifs":** Now comes the empowering part! For each "what if," ask yourself these questions:
    - **Is this "what if" based on facts or assumptions.** Are you catastrophizing or jumping to conclusions?
    - **What's the worst that could happen?** Is it really as bad as you imagine?
    - **What's the best that could happen?** Are there potential positive outcomes you haven't considered?
    - **What can I learn from this "what if"?** Can it help me make better choices in the future?

By challenging your "what ifs," you start to dismantle their power and create space for new possibilities.

THE BENEFITS OF THIS EXERCISE:

- **Increased Self-Awareness:** This exercise helps you become more aware of your thought patterns and the areas where fear and regret hold you back.
- **Shifting Perspectives:** By challenging your "what ifs," you start to see them in a new light, opening possibilities for growth and change.
- **Reduced Anxiety:** As you gain clarity and understanding, you'll likely experience a reduction in anxiety and worry.
- **Empowerment:** This exercise empowers you to take control of your thoughts and emotions, rather than being controlled by them.

IMPORTANT NOTE:

If you find that certain "what ifs" evoke intense emotions or trigger painful memories, be kind to yourself. You don't have to tackle everything at once. Consider seeking support from a therapist or counselor if you need additional guidance.

Remember, this exercise is a tool for self-discovery and growth. By facing your fears and regrets head-on, you pave the way for a more purposeful, fulfilling, and regret-free life.

Day 2: The Root of Fear and Regret

Yesterday, you took the brave step of acknowledging your "what ifs" – those nagging doubts and lingering regrets that have been holding you back. Today, we're going to dig a little deeper. We're going to explore the underlying causes of your fears and regrets, so you can understand them better and start to unravel their grip on your life.

Think of it as a bit of detective work. Just as a detective investigates a crime scene to uncover clues and motives, we're going to investigate your emotional landscape to uncover the sources of your fears and regrets. And trust me, this is not about dwelling on the negative. It's about gaining clarity, understanding your patterns, and laying the groundwork for lasting transformation.

THE ANATOMY OF FEAR

Fear is a complex emotion, one that has served humanity well throughout history. It's our built-in alarm system, designed to protect us from danger. However, in modern times, our fears often extend far beyond physical threats. We worry about our careers, our relationships, our finances, our health – the list goes on and on.

These fears, while sometimes valid, can easily spiral out of control if left unchecked. They can lead to chronic anxiety, self-doubt, and a reluctance to take risks. By understanding the root of your fears, you can start to disarm them and regain control of your life.

THE ORIGINS OF REGRET

Regret, like fear, is a universal human experience. We all have moments we wish we could do over, decisions we wish we had made differently, and opportunities we wish we had seized. But dwelling on these regrets can be incredibly damaging. It can lead to self-blame, shame, and a feeling of being stuck in the past.

Regret often stems from a perceived lack of control or agency. We feel like we've missed out on something important, and that feeling can be incredibly painful. But by examining the origins of your regrets, you can start to reframe them as opportunities for growth and learning.

UNCOVERING YOUR PATTERNS

The key to overcoming fear and regret is to understand their underlying causes. Are your fears rooted in past experiences, limiting beliefs, or societal expectations? Are your regrets driven by guilt, shame, or a fear of missing out?

By identifying your patterns, you'll gain valuable insights

into your emotional landscape. You'll see how your fears and regrets are interconnected, and how they might be influencing your decisions and behaviors. This self-awareness is the first step towards making positive changes.

YOUR FEAR AND REGRET JOURNAL

To help you uncover the root of your fears and regrets, I encourage you to create a journal dedicated to this exploration. In this journal, you'll record your thoughts, feelings, and any insights that arise as you delve deeper into your emotional landscape. It's a safe space for you to be honest with yourself and explore the complexities of your inner world.

Remember, this is not about dwelling on the negative. It's about gaining clarity, understanding your patterns, and laying the groundwork for transformation. By facing your fears and regrets head-on, you'll empower yourself to move forward with confidence, purpose, and a renewed sense of freedom.

UNDERSTANDING FEAR

Fear, my friend, is a complex and powerful emotion. It's a primal instinct, hardwired into our DNA to protect us from danger. It's the feeling that wells up in your chest when you're about to step out of your comfort zone, the tightness in your stomach when facing uncertainty, the racing thoughts that keep you awake at night.

But here's the thing: while fear can be a valuable ally, it can also become a formidable foe. It can warn us of real threats and keep us safe, but it can also morph into irrational anxieties that hold us back from reaching our full potential. Understanding the different types of fear and how they manifest is the first step to mastering them.

THE MANY FACES OF FEAR

Let's explore some of the most common fears that keep us trapped in the "what if" cycle:

1. **Fear of Failure:** This is the fear that we won't measure up, that we'll fall short, that we'll be judged or ridiculed. It can prevent us from trying new things, pursuing our dreams, or even speaking up for ourselves.
2. **Fear of Success:** Yes, success can be scary too! This fear often stems from the belief that we're not worthy of success or that it will bring unwanted changes and responsibilities. It can lead to self-sabotage, procrastination, or an inability to fully embrace our achievements.
3. **Fear of the Unknown:** This is the fear of uncertainty, change, and the unfamiliar. It can prevent us from taking risks, stepping outside our comfort zones, or embracing new opportunities.
4. **Fear of Rejection:** This is the fear of being judged, criticized, or ostracized by others. It can lead to people-pleasing behavior, a reluctance to express our true selves, and a fear of putting ourselves out there.
5. **Fear of Loss:** This is the fear of losing something or someone we value, such as a loved one, a job, or our health. It can lead to clinginess, anxiety, and an inability to enjoy the present moment.

HOW FEAR MANIFESTS

Fear can manifest in both physical and emotional ways. Physically, you might experience a racing heart, sweaty palms, shortness of breath, or even nausea. Emotionally, fear can lead to anxiety, worry, self-doubt, and even panic attacks.

But fear can also manifest in more subtle ways. It can show up as procrastination, avoidance, perfectionism, or people-pleasing behavior. It can cause you to overthink, second-guess yourself, and talk yourself out of taking action.

FEAR: PROTECTOR AND PARALYZER

Fear, in its purest form, is designed to protect us. When our ancestors faced real threats like wild animals or natural disasters, fear triggered the fight-or-flight response, which gave them the energy and focus to either confront the danger or escape to safety.

In our modern lives, we rarely face such immediate threats. However, our brains are still wired to react to perceived dangers, even if they're not life-threatening. This is why we can feel fear when giving a presentation, going on a first date, or starting a new business.

The problem is that when fear becomes excessive or irrational, it can paralyze us. Instead of protecting us, it prevents us from taking risks, pursuing our dreams, and living a full, authentic life.

UNDERSTANDING YOUR FEARS

The first step to mastering fear is to understand its origins. What are you truly afraid of? What are the underlying beliefs and assumptions that fuel your fears? Once you identify these root causes, you can start to challenge them and develop strategies for overcoming them.

The next section of this chapter will guide you through exercises to help you identify your specific fears and the emotions that accompany them. By understanding your fears, you'll be better equipped to face them head-on and take back control of your life.

THE NATURE OF REGRET

Regret is a complex emotion that can leave us feeling haunted by the past, trapped in a cycle of "what ifs" and "if onlys." But what exactly is regret, and where does it come from?

At its core, regret is the feeling of sadness, disappointment, or remorse that we experience when we believe we could have done something differently. It's a nagging sense that we've missed out on a better outcome or made a choice that we now wish we hadn't.

The Different Sources of Regret

Regret can stem from a variety of sources, each with its own unique flavor:

1. **Missed Opportunities:** This is the regret of inaction, the feeling that we didn't seize a chance when it was

presented to us. It's the "what if I had taken that job offer?" or the "if only I had spoken up" that can linger in our minds for years.

2. **Past Mistakes:** These are the regrets that arise from actions we took that we now wish we hadn't. It could be a hurtful comment we made, a relationship we sabotaged, or a decision that led to negative consequences.
3. **Wrong Decisions:** These regrets are tied to choices we made that turned out differently than we expected. They can be related to our career, relationships, finances, or any other area of life where we feel we've gone down the wrong path.

THE DOUBLE-EDGED SWORD OF REGRET

Regret can be a heavy burden to carry. It can lead to self-blame, shame, and a sense of powerlessness. When we dwell on our regrets, we get stuck in the past, unable to move forward and create a better future.

However, regret can also be a powerful catalyst for growth and transformation. When we examine our regrets with honesty and compassion, we can extract valuable lessons from them. We can learn about our values, our priorities, and the kind of choices we want to make in the future. Regret can serve as a wake-up call, motivating us to take action and make changes that align with our true selves.

REGRET AS A TEACHER

Think of regret as a teacher, offering you valuable feedback about your life choices. It's not about dwelling on the past or beating yourself up for mistakes. It's about using your regrets as a springboard for personal growth and positive change.

Here are some ways to reframe regret as a teacher:

1. **Identify the Lesson:** What can you learn from this experience? What did it teach you about your values, your needs, or your desires?
2. **Take Responsibility:** Acknowledge your role in the situation. What choices did you make that contributed to the outcome?
3. **Forgive Yourself:** Let go of self-blame and shame. We all make mistakes, and it's essential to forgive ourselves in order to move on.
4. **Make Amends (if possible):** If your regret involves hurting someone else, apologize and try to make things right.
5. **Create a Plan for Change:** Use the insights gained from your regret to create a plan for making different choices in the future.

FROM REGRET TO RESILIENCE

When we learn to embrace regret as a teacher, we can transform it from a source of pain into a source of power. We can use our regrets to fuel our growth, deepen our self-awareness, and make choices that align with our values and goals.

Remember, the past doesn't define us. It's what we do with our experiences that truly matters. By choosing to learn from our regrets, we can build resilience, cultivate wisdom, and create a future that we can be proud of.

The next time you find yourself dwelling on a regret, try to shift your focus from self-blame to self-compassion. Acknowledge your feelings, forgive yourself, and then ask yourself, "What can I learn from this?"

By reframing regret as a teacher, you can turn your past into a stepping stone towards a more fulfilling and purposeful future.

EXERCISE: FEAR AND REGRET JOURNAL

It's time to grab your journal and a pen. Don't worry, this isn't about perfect handwriting or eloquent prose. This is about raw honesty, deep reflection, and uncovering the truths that lie beneath your fears and regrets.

WHY A JOURNAL?

Putting pen to paper (or fingers to keyboard) has a unique power. It allows us to slow down, process our thoughts, and gain clarity on our emotions. Journaling can be a safe space to explore our inner world without judgment or fear of reprisal. It's like having a conversation with yourself, but with the added benefit of documenting your insights for future reference.

THE PURPOSE OF THIS EXERCISE

The Fear and Regret Journal is designed to help you:

1. **Identify Your Fears and Regrets:** By writing about specific instances of fear and regret, you'll gain a clearer understanding of what holds you back and what you wish you could change.
2. **Explore Your Emotions:** Delving into the emotions associated with these experiences will help you process them and move forward.
3. **Identify Patterns:** Look for recurring themes or triggers in your fears and regrets. This can reveal deeper beliefs or patterns of behavior that need to be addressed.
4. **Create a Roadmap for Change:** Your journal entries will serve as a valuable resource as you work through this book and beyond, helping you identify areas where you want to grow and change.

Instructions

1. **Choose a Specific Instance:** Think about a time when you experienced fear or regret. It could be a recent event or something from your past.
2. **Describe the Situation:** Write a detailed description of the situation, including what happened, who was involved, and what your role was.
3. **Explore Your Emotions:** What emotions did you feel at the time? Were you afraid, anxious, sad, angry, ashamed, or something else? Dig deep and describe your feelings as vividly as you can.
4. **Identify the Underlying Fear or Regret:** What was the specific fear or regret that was triggered by this situation? Were you afraid of failure, rejection, the

unknown? Did you regret a decision you made or an opportunity you missed?
5. **Reflect on the Impact:** How did this fear or regret impact your actions, your thoughts, your relationships, or your life in general? Be honest with yourself about the consequences of this experience.
6. **Look for Patterns:** Does this experience remind you of other times in your life when you've felt similar fears or regrets? Are there any recurring themes or triggers that you notice?

Example Journal Entry:

Situation: I was offered a promotion at work, but I declined it because I was afraid I wouldn't be able to handle the increased responsibility.

Emotions: I felt anxious, insecure, and unsure of myself. I was also disappointed in myself for not taking a chance.

Underlying Fear: Fear of failure. I was afraid I would mess up and embarrass myself in front of my colleagues and boss.

Impact: I missed out on a valuable opportunity for growth and advancement. I also started to doubt my abilities and question whether I was capable of taking on new challenges.

Pattern: I often hold myself back from trying new things because I'm afraid of failing.

TIPS FOR JOURNALING

- **Be Honest:** This journal is for your eyes only, so be honest with yourself about your thoughts and feelings.

There's no need to censor yourself or pretend to be someone you're not.
- **Don't Judge:** Approach your journal entries with curiosity and compassion. Avoid judging yourself or your experiences. Remember, everyone makes mistakes and experiences fear and regret.
- **Write Regularly:** Make journaling a regular practice. It can be helpful to set aside a specific time each day or week to write in your journal.
- **Explore Different Formats:** You can write in prose, create lists, draw pictures, or use whatever format feels most comfortable and expressive for you.

Remember, this journal is a tool for self-discovery and growth. By taking the time to explore your fears and regrets, you're taking an important step towards a more fulfilling and regret-free life.

Day 3: Changing Your Narrative

Have you ever caught yourself saying things like, "I'm not good enough," "I always mess things up," or "I'll never be able to do that"? We all have that inner voice, the one that whispers doubts, fears, and criticisms. It's like a constant soundtrack playing in the background of our lives, shaping our beliefs, our actions, and ultimately, our reality.

This inner dialogue, also known as self-talk, is incredibly powerful. It can either uplift us and propel us forward, or it can drag us down and hold us back. When we constantly tell ourselves negative stories, we start to believe them. We limit our potential, sabotage our goals, and reinforce our fears and regrets.

But here's the good news: you have the power to change your narrative. You can rewrite the script, silence the inner critic, and create a new story – one that empowers you, inspires you, and propels you toward your dreams.

This chapter is all about harnessing the power of words to transform your mindset. We'll explore how your thoughts and beliefs shape your reality, and you'll learn practical techniques for reframing negative self-talk into positive, empowering affirmations.

THE SCIENCE BEHIND SELF-TALK

Our brains are wired to believe the stories we tell ourselves, whether they're true or not. When we repeat negative thoughts, our brains create neural pathways that reinforce those beliefs, making them more likely to recur. It's like walking the same path over and over again – eventually, it becomes a well-worn groove.

But just as we can create negative neural pathways, we can also create positive ones. By consciously choosing to focus on empowering thoughts and affirmations, we can rewire our brains for success, happiness, and resilience.

Reframing: Your Key to a New Narrative

Reframing is a powerful technique for challenging negative thoughts and replacing them with more positive and realistic ones. It's like taking a picture and changing the frame – the picture itself doesn't change, but the way we perceive it does.

For example, instead of saying, "I'm a failure," you could reframe it as, "I'm learning and growing from this experience." Instead of saying, "I'm not good enough," you could say, "I'm worthy and capable."

Reframing isn't about denying reality or pretending everything is perfect. It's about choosing to focus on the positive aspects of a situation and looking for opportunities for growth and learning.

YOUR WORDS, YOUR POWER

The words you use to describe yourself and your experiences matter. They shape your beliefs, influence your emotions, and impact your actions. By consciously choosing to use positive, empowering language, you can transform your mindset and create a new narrative that supports your goals and dreams.

In the exercise for this chapter, you'll start to practice reframing your negative thoughts into positive affirmations. This is a simple yet powerful tool that can have a profound impact on your life. By repeating these affirmations daily, you'll gradually rewire your brain to focus on the positive and overcome the self-doubt that holds you back.

Remember, your words have power. Use them wisely to create the life you desire.

THE POWER OF SELF-TALK

Ever caught yourself thinking, "I'm not good enough," or "I always mess things up"? These aren't just fleeting thoughts; they're powerful stories that we tell ourselves about who we are and what we're capable of. And here's the kicker: our brains believe the stories we feed them, whether they're true or not.

This inner dialogue, also known as self-talk, is like a constant narrator in the movie of our lives. It provides commentary, interprets events, and shapes our perceptions. But just like a movie narrator, our self-talk isn't always reliable. It can be overly critical, pessimistic, and downright mean.

Negative self-talk is like a broken record, playing the same tired tunes of inadequacy, fear, and regret. It tells us we're not smart enough, talented enough, or worthy enough. It whispers doubts in our ears and convinces us to play it safe, stay small, and avoid taking risks.

But here's the thing: these negative stories are not facts. They are simply thoughts—often distorted and exaggerated versions of reality. Yet, when we believe these stories, they become self-fulfilling prophecies.

HOW NEGATIVE SELF-TALK PERPETUATES FEAR AND REGRET

Imagine this: You're about to give a presentation at work. Your heart is pounding, your palms are sweaty, and your mind is racing with thoughts like, "I'm going to mess this up," or "They're all going to think I'm an idiot."

These negative thoughts trigger a stress response in your body. Your cortisol levels spike, your breathing becomes shallow, and your focus narrows. You start to doubt your preparation, stumble over your words, and forget important points. Afterward, you berate yourself for your perceived failure, reinforcing the negative story that you're not good enough.

This is how negative self-talk perpetuates fear and regret. It creates a self-doubt spiral that keeps us from taking action, pursuing our goals, and reaching our full potential. We become so afraid of failure or rejection that we don't even try. And when we do take a chance and things don't go as planned, we beat ourselves up with regret, further fueling the negative self-talk.

THE VICIOUS CYCLE OF SELF-SABOTAGE

Negative self-talk can also lead to self-sabotage. We may unconsciously engage in behaviors that confirm our negative beliefs, such as procrastinating on important tasks, avoiding challenges, or pushing away supportive people.

For example, if you believe you're not worthy of love, you might subconsciously sabotage your relationships by picking fights, pushing your partner away, or settling for less than you deserve.

The good news is that you have the power to change your inner dialogue. You can rewrite the script, silence the inner critic, and cultivate a more positive and empowering mindset. This is where the 30-day challenge comes in. Throughout this book, you'll learn practical strategies to challenge negative self-talk, reframe your thoughts, and build a stronger sense of self-belief.

FROM SELF-DOUBT TO SELF-BELIEF

Imagine what your life could be like if your inner dialogue was your biggest cheerleader instead of your harshest critic. What if, instead of focusing on your flaws, you focused on your strengths? Instead of dwelling on past mistakes, you learned from them and moved forward? Instead of letting fear hold you back, you embraced it as an opportunity for growth?

This is the transformative power of positive self-talk. It can boost your confidence, increase your motivation, and empower you to take action towards your goals. It can help you break free from the cycle of fear and regret and start living a life that is aligned with your purpose and values.

The journey to positive self-talk isn't always easy, but it's worth it. It's a commitment to yourself, your well-being, and your dreams. And it all starts with recognizing the power of your thoughts and choosing to tell yourself a new, more empowering story.

REFRAMING YOUR THOUGHTS

Alright, let's get real for a moment. How many times have you caught yourself thinking, "I'm not good enough," "I'll never succeed," or "Why do I always mess things up?"

These negative thoughts are like little gremlins whispering doubts and fears into your ear. They can chip away at your confidence, hold you back from taking action, and leave you feeling stuck in a rut. But here's the good news: you don't have to be a victim of your own thoughts. You have the power to reframe them, turning negativity into fuel for growth and empowerment.

Think of your thoughts as a garden. Just like weeds can choke out beautiful flowers, negative thoughts can overshadow your potential and stifle your joy. But with a little effort, you can pull those weeds, plant seeds of positivity, and cultivate a vibrant and flourishing mental landscape.

WHAT IS REFRAMING?

Reframing is simply the act of shifting your perspective. It's about looking at a situation, thought, or belief from a different angle, one that's more positive, empowering, and productive.

Let's say you make a mistake at work. Your initial thought might be, "I'm such an idiot. I always screw things up." This negative thought can spiral into feelings of shame, self-doubt, and even despair. But what if you reframed it? Instead of dwelling on the mistake, you could say to yourself, "Everyone makes mistakes. This is an opportunity for me to learn and grow."

By reframing the situation, you've taken away its power to define you. You've shifted your focus from self-blame to self-improvement. And that, my friend, is a game-changer.

THE BENEFITS OF REFRAMING

Reframing isn't about denying reality or pretending that everything is perfect. It's about choosing to focus on the positive aspects of a situation, even when things are tough. When you reframe negative thoughts, you:

- **Reduce stress and anxiety:** Negative thoughts can trigger a stress response in your body. Reframing helps you calm down and approach challenges with a clearer head.
- **Increase confidence:** When you focus on your strengths and capabilities, your self-belief grows.
- **Improve problem-solving:** Reframing opens up new possibilities and solutions that may have been hidden by negativity.

- **Boost resilience:** You become better equipped to handle setbacks and bounce back from adversity.

Techniques for Reframing

There are many different ways to reframe negative thoughts. Here are a few simple yet effective techniques you can start using today:

1. **Challenge the Thought:** Ask yourself if the thought is truly accurate or if it's just a fear-based assumption.
2. **Look for Evidence:** Gather evidence that supports a more positive interpretation of the situation.
3. **Focus on Solutions:** Instead of dwelling on the problem, brainstorm possible solutions or actions you can take.
4. **Practice Gratitude:** Shift your focus to the things you're grateful for in your life.
5. **Use Humor:** Sometimes, a little humor can help diffuse a negative situation and put things in perspective.
6. **Talk to a Supportive Friend:** Sharing your thoughts with someone you trust can provide a fresh perspective and valuable support.
7. **Use Affirmations:** Repeat positive affirmations that counter your negative thoughts.

Remember: Reframing is a skill, and like any skill, it takes practice. Don't get discouraged if you don't see results immediately. Keep practicing, be patient with yourself, and celebrate your progress.

By consistently reframing your thoughts, you'll create a

more positive and empowering mindset. You'll build the resilience to overcome challenges, the confidence to pursue your dreams, and the clarity to make choices that align with your purpose. So let's ditch those negative gremlins and start cultivating a garden of positivity within our minds. The power to transform your life is in your hands.

EXERCISE: AFFIRMATION JOURNALING

Grab your journal, friend, because it's time for a powerful exercise that can transform your mindset and propel you towards your dreams. We're going to dive into the world of affirmations and rewrite the negative scripts that have been holding you back.

WHAT ARE AFFIRMATIONS?

Affirmations are short, powerful statements that you repeat to yourself regularly. They're like little mantras that you program into your subconscious mind, helping to shift your beliefs, boost your confidence, and attract positive experiences into your life.

Think of affirmations as seeds you plant in the fertile soil of your mind. With consistent watering and nurturing, these seeds can grow into beautiful, thriving plants—new beliefs, habits, and possibilities.

WHY AFFIRMATIONS WORK

Affirmations work by tapping into the power of neuroplasticity, which is the brain's ability to change and reorganize itself by forming new neural connections. When you repeat affirmations, you're essentially rewiring your brain to focus on the positive aspects of yourself and your life.

This isn't just wishful thinking or positive vibes. Science backs it up. Studies have shown that affirmations can reduce stress, increase self-esteem, improve performance, and even change the structure of our brains.

CRAFTING YOUR AFFIRMATIONS

Now, let's get personal. Remember those fears and regrets you identified on Day 1 and Day 2? We're going to use them as fuel to create affirmations that directly counter those negative thoughts.

Here are some tips for crafting effective affirmations:

1. **Make them personal:** Use "I" statements and speak to yourself as if you're already living the life you desire. For example, instead of saying "I hope to be confident," say "I am confident and capable."
2. **Keep them positive:** Avoid using negative words like "don't," "can't," or "won't." Focus on what you *want* to achieve, not what you want to avoid.
3. **Use the present tense:** Speak as if your desired outcome is already happening. This helps to trick your mind into believing it's true and making it a reality.
4. **Make them specific:** The more specific your affirmations, the more powerful they become. For example, instead of saying "I am successful," say "I am a

successful entrepreneur who makes a positive impact on the world."
5. **Infuse them with emotion:** Affirmations that evoke positive emotions are more likely to stick. Use words and phrases that make you feel excited, empowered, and inspired.

Examples of Affirmations to Counter Fears and Regrets:

- **Fear of Failure:** "I embrace challenges as opportunities for growth."
- **Fear of Rejection:** "I am worthy of love and acceptance."
- **Regret Over Past Mistakes:** "I have learned from my past and I am moving forward with strength and wisdom."
- **Self-Doubt:** "I trust in my abilities and I am capable of achieving my goals."
- **Lack of Confidence:** "I am confident in my own skin and I radiate self-assurance."

YOUR DAILY AFFIRMATION PRACTICE

Once you've crafted your affirmations, it's time to put them into practice. Here's a simple routine you can follow:

1. **Choose a Time:** Pick a time each day when you can dedicate a few minutes to your affirmations. This could be first thing in the morning, during your lunch break, or before bed.

2. **Find a Quiet Space:** Settle into a comfortable position where you won't be interrupted.
3. **Repeat Your Affirmations:** Read your affirmations aloud or silently, focusing on the meaning of each word. Repeat them several times, allowing the words to sink into your subconscious.
4. **Visualize:** As you repeat your affirmations, visualize yourself living the life you desire. See yourself achieving your goals, overcoming your fears, and embracing your purpose.
5. **Feel the Emotions:** Allow yourself to feel the emotions associated with your affirmations. Feel the joy, excitement, confidence, or gratitude that comes with living your best life.

Remember, consistency is key. The more you repeat your affirmations, the more powerful they become. Make them a part of your daily routine and watch as they transform your mindset and your life.

Affirmation Journaling Tips:

- **Write Them Down:** Write your affirmations in your journal each day. This helps to solidify them in your mind and allows you to track your progress.
- **Get Creative:** Don't be afraid to experiment with different formats. You can write your affirmations as a list, a poem, or even a song.
- **Make it Fun:** Add some flair to your journal with

colorful pens, stickers, or drawings. The more enjoyable the process, the more likely you are to stick with it.

Remember, this is your personal journey. Choose affirmations that resonate with you and adapt your practice to fit your lifestyle and preferences. The most important thing is to make it a habit and to trust in the power of your words to create the life you desire.

TECHNIQUES FOR REFRAMING

There are many different ways to reframe negative thoughts. Here are a few simple yet effective techniques you can start using today:

1. **Challenge the Thought:** Ask yourself if the thought is truly accurate or if it's just a fear-based assumption.
2. **Look for Evidence:** Gather evidence that supports a more positive interpretation of the situation.
3. **Focus on Solutions:** Instead of dwelling on the problem, brainstorm possible solutions or actions you can take.
4. **Practice Gratitude:** Shift your focus to the things you're grateful for in your life.
5. **Use Humor:** Sometimes, a little humor can help diffuse a negative situation and put things in perspective.
6. **Talk to a Supportive Friend:** Sharing your thoughts with someone you trust can provide a fresh perspective and valuable support.

7. **Use Affirmations:** Repeat positive affirmations that counter your negative thoughts.

Remember: Reframing is a skill, and like any skill, it takes practice. Don't get discouraged if you don't see results immediately. Keep practicing, be patient with yourself, and celebrate your progress.

By consistently reframing your thoughts, you'll create a more positive and empowering mindset. You'll build the resilience to overcome challenges, the confidence to pursue your dreams, and the clarity to make choices that align with your purpose. So let's ditch those negative gremlins and start cultivating a garden of positivity within our minds. The power to transform your life is in your hands.

EXERCISE: AFFIRMATION JOURNALING

Grab your journal, friend, because it's time for a powerful exercise that can transform your mindset and propel you towards your dreams. We're going to dive into the world of affirmations and rewrite the negative scripts that have been holding you back.

WHAT ARE AFFIRMATIONS?

Affirmations are short, powerful statements that you repeat to yourself regularly. They're like little mantras that you program into your subconscious mind, helping to shift your beliefs, boost your confidence, and attract positive experiences into your life.

Think of affirmations as seeds you plant in the fertile soil of your mind. With consistent watering and nurturing, these seeds can grow into beautiful, thriving plants—new beliefs, habits, and possibilities.

WHY AFFIRMATIONS WORK

Affirmations work by tapping into the power of neuroplasticity, which is the brain's ability to change and reorganize itself by forming new neural connections. When you repeat affirmations, you're essentially rewiring your brain to focus on the positive aspects of yourself and your life.

This isn't just wishful thinking or positive vibes. Science backs it up. Studies have shown that affirmations can reduce stress, increase self-esteem, improve performance, and even change the structure of our brains.

Crafting Your Affirmations

Now, let's get personal. Remember those fears and regrets you identified on Day 1 and Day 2? We're going to use them as fuel to create affirmations that directly counter those negative thoughts.

Here are some tips for crafting effective affirmations:

1. **Make them personal:** Use "I" statements and speak to yourself as if you're already living the life you desire. For example, instead of saying "I hope to be confident," say "I am confident and capable."
2. **Keep them positive:** Avoid using negative words like "don't," "can't," or "won't." Focus on what you *want* to achieve, not what you want to avoid.

3. **Use the present tense:** Speak as if your desired outcome is already happening. This helps to trick your mind into believing it's true and making it a reality.
4. **Make them specific:** The more specific your affirmations, the more powerful they become. For example, instead of saying "I am successful," say "I am a successful entrepreneur who makes a positive impact on the world."
5. **Infuse them with emotion:** Affirmations that evoke positive emotions are more likely to stick. Use words and phrases that make you feel excited, empowered, and inspired.

Examples of Affirmations to Counter Fears and Regrets:

- **Fear of Failure:** "I embrace challenges as opportunities for growth."
- **Fear of Rejection:** "I am worthy of love and acceptance."
- **Regret Over Past Mistakes:** "I have learned from my past and I am moving forward with strength and wisdom."
- **Self-Doubt:** "I trust in my abilities and I am capable of achieving my goals."
- **Lack of Confidence:** "I am confident in my own skin and I radiate self-assurance."

Your Daily Affirmation Practice

Once you've crafted your affirmations, it's time to put them into practice. Here's a simple routine you can follow:

1. **Choose a Time:** Pick a time each day when you can dedicate a few minutes to your affirmations. This could be first thing in the morning, during your lunch break, or before bed.
2. **Find a Quiet Space:** Settle into a comfortable position where you won't be interrupted.
3. **Repeat Your Affirmations:** Read your affirmations aloud or silently, focusing on the meaning of each word. Repeat them several times, allowing the words to sink into your subconscious.
4. **Visualize:** As you repeat your affirmations, visualize yourself living the life you desire. See yourself achieving your goals, overcoming your fears, and embracing your purpose.
5. **Feel the Emotions:** Allow yourself to feel the emotions associated with your affirmations. Feel the joy, excitement, confidence, or gratitude that comes with living your best life.

Remember, consistency is key. The more you repeat your affirmations, the more powerful they become. Make them a part of your daily routine and watch as they transform your mindset and your life.

Affirmation Journaling Tips:

- **Write Them Down:** Write your affirmations in your

journal each day. This helps to solidify them in your mind and allows you to track your progress.
- **Get Creative:** Don't be afraid to experiment with different formats. You can write your affirmations as a list, a poem, or even a song.
- **Make it Fun:** Add some flair to your journal with colorful pens, stickers, or drawings. The more enjoyable the process, the more likely you are to stick with it.

Remember, this is your personal journey. Choose affirmations that resonate with you and adapt your practice to fit your lifestyle and preferences. The most important thing is to make it a habit and to trust in the power of your words to create the life you desire.

Day 4: The Courage to Act

If fear and regret are the anchors that hold us back, then action is the wind that fills our sails and propels us forward. But how do we move from a state of inaction, fueled by "what ifs," to one of bold, purposeful action? It all starts with cultivating courage.

Courage isn't the absence of fear; it's the willingness to act *despite* fear. It's the decision to step outside our comfort zones, even when our hearts are pounding, and our minds are racing with doubt.

Think back to a time when you felt truly alive, when you were fully engaged in the present moment and pursuing something that mattered to you. Chances are, you were acting courageously, pushing past your fears to embrace a new experience, challenge yourself, or make a meaningful contribution.

The truth is, we all have courage within us. It's a muscle that can be strengthened and developed with practice. And the more we use it, the easier it becomes to take bold action, even in the face of uncertainty or fear.

In this chapter, we'll explore the relationship between courage and action. We'll discuss why taking action is essential for overcoming fear and regret, and we'll provide practical strategies for cultivating the courage to step out of your comfort zone and start living your purpose.

FROM INACTION TO ACTION: BREAKING THE CYCLE

Fear often leads to inaction. When we're afraid of failure, rejection, or the unknown, it's easy to stay stuck in a state of paralysis, endlessly analyzing our options and dwelling on potential risks.

But inaction is a breeding ground for regret. When we look back on our lives, we're more likely to regret the things we didn't do than the things we did.

The key to breaking this cycle is to take action, even if it's just a small step. Each action you take builds momentum, confidence, and resilience. It reinforces the belief that you are capable of achieving your goals and living a life of purpose.

EMBRACING IMPERFECTION: PROGRESS OVER PERFECTION

One of the biggest obstacles to taking action is the fear of not being perfect. We worry about making mistakes, looking foolish, or not living up to our own (often unrealistic) expectations.

But perfection is an illusion. Everyone makes mistakes, and even the most successful people experience setbacks and failures along the way. The key is to embrace imperfection as a natural part of the learning process.

When we focus on progress instead of perfection, we give ourselves permission to take risks, experiment, and learn from our experiences. We become more resilient in the face of challenges and less afraid of failing.

THE "WHY NOT?" MINDSET

Instead of asking yourself, "What if I fail?" start asking, "Why not me?" This simple shift in perspective can empower you to take action and embrace the opportunities that life presents.

Remember, every successful person started somewhere. They had doubts, fears, and insecurities just like you. But they chose to act despite those feelings, and they eventually achieved their dreams.

So, why not you? Why not now?

In the exercise for this chapter, we'll challenge you to take that first step toward overcoming your fears and regrets. It's time to move from "what if" to "why not?" and start living the life you were meant to live.

FROM INACTION TO ACTION

Let's be honest, fear can be a real drag. It has a sneaky way of whispering doubts in our ears, casting shadows on our dreams, and ultimately keeping us stuck in a cycle of inaction. But here's the thing: fear doesn't have to be the boss of you.

You can learn to dance with it, harness its energy, and use it as a springboard for action.

THE PROCRASTINATION PARADOX

Have you ever found yourself putting off a task you know you need to do? Maybe it's starting a new project, having a difficult conversation, or taking a leap of faith toward a goal. You tell yourself you'll do it later, but "later" never seems to come.

This is the procrastination paradox: we procrastinate on the very things that could bring us closer to our dreams, simply because we're afraid of what might happen if we try. We fear failure, rejection, judgment, or even success itself. So instead of taking action, we stay stuck in a comfortable but stagnant state.

Procrastination is often fueled by a desire to avoid discomfort. We tell ourselves that we'll wait until we feel more confident, have more time, or know more about the situation. But here's the truth: those perfect conditions rarely exist. The longer we wait, the more our fears solidify and the harder it becomes to take action.

THE SMALL STEPS STRATEGY

So, how do we break free from the chains of fear and procrastination? The answer lies in the power of small, consistent steps.

Think of it like this: imagine you're standing at the base of a mountain, gazing up at the daunting peak. The thought of climbing the entire mountain in one go can be overwhelming and paralyzing. But what if you focused on taking one step at a time? What if you broke down the climb into smaller, more manageable chunks?

The same principle applies to overcoming fear and procrastination. Instead of focusing on the enormity of your goals, break them down into bite-sized tasks that feel less intimidating. This could involve:

- **Setting a timer:** Commit to working on a task for just 15-20 minutes without distractions. You'll often find that once you get started, you'll gain momentum and want to continue.
- **Identifying the next small step:** Ask yourself, "What's the next logical action I can take to move closer to my goal?" This could be as simple as sending an email, doing some research, or outlining a plan.
- **Creating a daily action list:** Write down 3-5 tasks that you can realistically accomplish each day. This creates a sense of progress and helps you avoid feeling overwhelmed.

THE SNOWBALL EFFECT

As you consistently take small steps, you'll start to notice a snowball effect. Each action builds upon the last, creating momentum and boosting your confidence. The more you act, the less power your fears have over you.

It's like pushing a boulder up a hill. At first, it feels incredibly heavy and difficult to budge. But with each push, it gains a little more momentum. Eventually, the boulder starts rolling on its own, gaining speed and power as it goes.

The same thing happens when we take action despite our fears. Each step we take gives us the courage to take another, and

before we know it, we're moving forward with a force that we never thought possible.

THE POWER OF CONSISTENCY

Consistency is key to overcoming fear and procrastination. It's not about taking massive leaps every day; it's about making small, sustainable progress that compounds over time. Think of it like exercising. You don't get in shape by going to the gym once and lifting a ton of weight. You get in shape by showing up consistently, even when you don't feel like it.

So, commit to taking action every day, even if it's just for a few minutes. Set a timer, make a plan, and get started. You'll be amazed at how much you can accomplish when you harness the power of small, consistent steps.

Remember, fear is not the enemy; it's a messenger. It's telling you that you're about to step outside your comfort zone, that you're about to grow and expand. So, embrace the fear, acknowledge it, and then take action anyway. That's where the magic happens.

EMBRACING IMPERFECTION

Let's be real for a moment: nobody's perfect. Not you, not me, not even the most successful people on the planet. Yet, we're often bombarded with messages that suggest otherwise. We scroll through social media and see carefully curated highlight reels, compare ourselves to others, and feel inadequate when we don't measure up.

This relentless pursuit of perfection is a trap. It's a mirage that keeps us chasing an unattainable ideal, leading to procrastination, anxiety, and a crippling fear of failure. It's time to break free from this illusion and embrace the messy, beautiful reality of imperfection.

THE PERFECTIONISM PARADOX

Perfectionism might seem like a noble pursuit, but it often backfires. Striving for flawlessness can paralyze us, preventing us from taking action for fear of not being good enough. We overthink, overanalyze, and second-guess ourselves, missing out on opportunities and experiences that could enrich our lives.

Perfectionism can also lead to burnout and overwhelm. When we set impossibly high standards for ourselves, we create a constant state of pressure and stress. We become our own worst critics, berating ourselves for every mistake or perceived flaw.

But what if I told you that your imperfections are not your weaknesses, but your greatest strengths? What if I told you that embracing your flaws is the key to unlocking your full potential?

THE BEAUTY OF IMPERFECTION

Imperfection is not a sign of failure; it's a sign of humanity. It's what makes us unique, relatable, and capable of growth. Embracing our imperfections allows us to be authentic, to learn from our mistakes, and to connect with others on a deeper level.

When we let go of the need to be perfect, we free ourselves to take risks, try new things, and pursue our passions without fear of judgment or failure. We become more resilient, adaptable, and creative. We open ourselves up to a world of possibilities that were previously out of reach.

Think about your favorite artists, musicians, or writers. Are their works perfect? Of course not! Yet, it's their imperfections, their unique quirks and flaws, that make their work so captivating and relatable.

The same is true for you. Your imperfections are not obstacles to overcome, but integral parts of who you are. They are the brushstrokes that create the masterpiece of your life.

LEARNING FROM MISTAKES

One of the most powerful gifts of imperfection is the opportunity to learn and grow from our mistakes. When we strive for perfection, we fear making mistakes. But when we embrace imperfection, we see mistakes as valuable feedback, as stepping stones on our path to success.

Think about a time when you made a mistake. Did it teach you something? Did it help you grow? Chances are, the answer is yes. Every mistake is an opportunity to learn, to adapt, and to become a better version of yourself.

Embracing mistakes doesn't mean being careless or reckless. It means accepting that we are human and that we will inevitably make mistakes along the way. It means having the courage to learn from those mistakes and use them as fuel for growth.

PROGRESS, NOT PERFECTION

The key to living a regret-free life is not to avoid mistakes altogether, but to focus on progress, not perfection. It's about taking action, learning as you go, and celebrating every step forward, no matter how small.

Remember, every expert was once a beginner. Every successful person has faced countless setbacks and failures. The difference is that they didn't let those setbacks define them. They learned from them, grew from them, and kept moving forward.

So, embrace your imperfections. Embrace your mistakes. Embrace your journey. It's in those moments of vulnerability and authenticity that you'll discover your true strength, your true resilience, and your true potential.

EXERCISE: "NO MORE WHAT IFS" CHALLENGE

Today, we're taking a bold step towards transforming those lingering "what ifs" into "why nots?" We're going to face our fears head-on and take action.

Think of it as a friendly nudge, a gentle push, a loving kick in the pants (if you need it!). It's time to move beyond the endless loop of hypotheticals and into the realm of real-life experience.

THE POWER OF SMALL, BRAVE ACTIONS

You might be thinking, "But what if I fail?" or "What if it doesn't work out?" That's okay. Fear is a natural part of the process. But remember, we're not aiming for perfection here. We're aiming for progress.

The "No More What If" Challenge isn't about making grand gestures or taking massive leaps. It's about starting small. Think of it as building a muscle. Just like you wouldn't start a workout routine by lifting the heaviest weights, you don't need to start your journey to "no more what ifs" by tackling your biggest fear.

Instead, choose one small, brave action that you've been putting off due to fear or regret. This could be anything from:

- **Applying for a job:** That dream position you've been eyeing but haven't had the courage to go for? Today's the day to hit "submit" on that application.
- **Having a difficult conversation:** Is there someone you need to talk to, but you've been avoiding it because it feels uncomfortable? Pick up the phone or schedule a meeting.
- **Starting a creative project:** Have you always wanted to write a book, paint a picture, or start a blog? Today's the day to put pen to paper, brush to canvas, or fingers to keyboard.

- **Taking a class or workshop:** Is there a skill you've been wanting to learn or a hobby you've been wanting to explore? Sign up for that class or workshop today.
- **Trying something new:** Maybe it's trying a new food, visiting a new place, or starting a new fitness routine. Step outside your comfort zone and expand your horizons.

It doesn't matter what you choose, as long as it's something that pushes you slightly beyond your comfort zone and aligns with your values and goals. Remember, even the smallest step can lead to significant change.

TAKING THE PLUNGE

Once you've chosen your "No More What If" Challenge, it's time to take action. Set a deadline for yourself (today, this week, or this month), and commit to following through. Don't let fear or doubt hold you back.

Here are a few tips to help you take the plunge:

- **Acknowledge your fear:** It's okay to feel scared. Acknowledge the fear, but don't let it control you.
- **Focus on the positive:** What are the potential benefits of taking this action? Visualize the positive outcomes.
- **Prepare and plan:** If necessary, take some time to prepare or plan for your challenge. This could involve researching, gathering information, or practicing your skills.
- **Tell someone:** Share your challenge with a supportive

friend, family member, or mentor. Having someone to cheer you on can make a big difference.
- **Reward yourself:** Once you've completed your challenge, take the time to celebrate your accomplishment.

LEARNING FROM THE EXPERIENCE

No matter what the outcome of your challenge, remember that it's a learning opportunity. If it goes well, celebrate your success and build on it. If it doesn't go as planned, don't beat yourself up. Instead, reflect on what you can learn from the experience and how you can apply those lessons to future challenges.

The "No More What If" Challenge is not just a one-time event. It's a mindset shift, a commitment to taking action and moving forward, even in the face of fear and uncertainty.

By consistently challenging yourself to step outside your comfort zone, you'll gradually build your confidence, resilience, and sense of empowerment. You'll start to see that you are capable of so much more than you ever thought possible.

So, what are you waiting for? Choose your challenge, take the plunge, and start living a life of "no more what ifs." Your future self will thank you.

Day 5: Facing Your Fears

Remember that scene in every adventure movie where the hero stands at the base of a daunting mountain? The wind howls, snow whips around, and the peak seems impossibly distant. Their heart pounds with a mix of fear and excitement. But they know they must face this challenge head-on. Why? Because on the other side of that mountain lies their destiny.

Your fears are your personal mountains. They loom large, casting shadows of doubt and uncertainty. They whisper tales of failure, rejection, and pain. And just like that mountain climber, you might feel a knot in your stomach every time you think about facing them.

But here's the thing: facing your fears is not about being fearless. It's about acknowledging the fear, feeling it fully, and then taking action in spite of it. It's about recognizing that fear is not a stop sign; it's a signpost pointing you towards growth.

In this chapter, we're going to equip you with the tools and strategies to climb your personal mountain. We'll help you understand the nature of fear, break it down into manageable

steps, and build the courage to take action. We'll guide you through a process called the "Fear Ladder," a technique that
gradually exposes you to your fears, allowing you to build confidence and resilience with each step.

You might be wondering, "What's on the other side of my mountain?" The answer is simple: freedom. Freedom from the shackles of fear, the chains of regret, and the "what ifs" that have held you back. On the other side of your mountain lies a life of purpose, passion, and possibility. A life where you're no longer a victim of your circumstances but the empowered creator of your own destiny.

So, are you ready to lace up your boots, grab your gear, and start climbing? Let's conquer those fears together, one step at a time. Remember, you are not alone. I'll be right there with you, cheering you on every step of the way.

THE FEAR LADDER

Imagine fear as a towering ladder. At the bottom rung are the small, manageable anxieties we face every day – maybe it's speaking up in a meeting or trying a new recipe. As we climb higher, the rungs represent progressively more daunting challenges – perhaps starting a business, asking someone out, or traveling alone. At the very top is our biggest, most paralyzing fear.

Now, imagine trying to jump straight to the top of that ladder. Terrifying, right? Most of us would freeze, overwhelmed by the sheer height and potential for a painful fall. That's why we need a different approach – one that allows us to climb gradually, building confidence and resilience with each step.

This is where the concept of the fear ladder comes in. It's a powerful tool that helps us break down our fears into smaller, more manageable steps. Instead of trying to tackle our biggest fear head-on, we start with the smallest, least intimidating step and gradually work our way up.

HOW DOES THE FEAR LADDER WORK?

The fear ladder is based on the principle of exposure therapy, a proven method for overcoming anxiety and phobias. The idea is to gradually expose ourselves to the things we fear in a controlled and safe environment.

Here's how it works:

1. **Identify Your Fear:** What is the specific fear you want to overcome? Be specific and concrete. For example, instead of saying "I'm afraid of public speaking," you might say, "I'm afraid of giving a presentation to my colleagues."
2. **Create Your Ladder:** Break down your fear into a series of increasingly challenging steps. Start with the smallest, most manageable step and gradually work your way up to the most challenging. For example, your fear ladder for public speaking might look like this:
    - Step 1: Practice giving a presentation to myself in the mirror.
    - Step 2: Give a presentation to a trusted friend or family member.

- Step 3: Record myself giving a presentation and watch it back.
- Step 4: Give a presentation to a small group of friends or colleagues.
- Step 5: Give a presentation to a larger group of colleagues.

3. **Climb the Ladder:** Start with the first step on your ladder and practice it repeatedly until your anxiety decreases. Once you feel comfortable with that step, move on to the next one. Continue climbing the ladder, one step at a time, until you reach the top.
4. **Celebrate Your Progress:** Acknowledge and celebrate each step you take. Remember, progress – not perfection – is the goal.

THE SCIENCE BEHIND THE FEAR LADDER

The fear ladder works because it taps into a process called habituation. When we repeatedly expose ourselves to something we fear, our brains gradually become less reactive to it. This is because our brains are designed to adapt to new situations and stimuli.

Think about it this way: the first time you hear a loud noise, you might jump or feel startled. But if you hear that same noise over and over again, you'll eventually get used to it and it won't bother you as much. The same principle applies to fear. By gradually exposing ourselves to our fears, we essentially teach our brains that they're not as dangerous as we initially thought.

PRACTICAL TIPS FOR CLIMBING YOUR FEAR LADDER

- **Start small:** Don't tackle your biggest fear right away. Begin with a step that feels challenging but doable.
- **Be consistent:** Practice each step on your ladder regularly. The more you expose yourself to your fear, the faster you'll overcome it.
- **Focus on your breathing:** When you feel anxious, take a few deep breaths to calm your nervous system.
- **Challenge negative thoughts:** When those "what ifs" creep in, challenge them with evidence and positive affirmations.
- **Celebrate your wins:** Acknowledge and celebrate each step you take on your fear ladder.

Remember, climbing the fear ladder is not about eliminating fear altogether. It's about learning to manage it and use it as a catalyst for growth. As you face your fears head-on, you'll discover that you're stronger and more capable than you ever imagined.

The fear ladder is a powerful tool for overcoming fear and regret. It's a gradual, step-by-step approach that allows us to confront our anxieties in a safe and controlled way. By climbing our fear ladders, we can break free from the limitations that hold us back and live a life of greater freedom, purpose, and joy.

BUILDING COURAGE MUSCLES

Imagine courage as a muscle, one that grows stronger with each flex, each challenge you face head-on. Every time you step outside your comfort zone, you're essentially doing a rep in the gym of life, building your resilience and confidence. Let's dive into how facing your fears actually strengthens your courage muscles.

FACING FEARS: THE KEY TO GROWTH

Think about a time when you did something that scared you. Maybe you gave a presentation in front of a large group, started a new job, or even just spoke up when you usually stay quiet. Remember the feeling of accomplishment, the surge of confidence that came after? That's your courage muscle flexing!

Facing our fears isn't about becoming fearless; it's about learning to act *despite* fear. It's about recognizing that fear is often just a signal, not a stop sign. When we understand that we can feel fear and still move forward, we begin to see challenges as opportunities for growth, not insurmountable obstacles.

Each time you confront a fear, you're essentially training your brain to respond differently. You're rewiring your neural pathways to create new associations between the feared situation and a sense of accomplishment. This strengthens your courage muscle, making it easier to face similar challenges in the future.

THE RESILIENCE FACTOR

Facing our fears not only builds courage, but it also cultivates resilience – that remarkable ability to bounce back from setbacks and challenges. Think of resilience as the shock absorber of your emotional well-being. It allows you to navigate life's inevitable bumps and detours without getting derailed.

When we avoid our fears, we rob ourselves of the opportunity to develop resilience. We create a false sense of security, but we also miss out on the chance to learn, grow, and become stronger.

Every time you face a fear and come out on the other side, you're sending a powerful message to yourself: "I can handle this. I am capable." This reinforces your belief in yourself and your ability to overcome challenges, which in turn fuels your resilience.

CONFIDENCE: THE BYPRODUCT OF COURAGE

As you continue to face your fears and build resilience, something magical happens: your confidence soars. You start to trust yourself more. You believe in your abilities. You know that even if things don't go as planned, you can handle it.

Confidence isn't about being arrogant or believing you're perfect. It's about having a realistic assessment of your strengths and weaknesses, acknowledging your fears, and still believing in your ability to succeed. It's about knowing that you have what it takes to navigate life's challenges, no matter what comes your way.

PRACTICAL TIPS FOR BUILDING COURAGE MUSCLES

1. **Start Small:** Don't try to tackle your biggest fear right away. Begin with small, manageable steps. This could be speaking up in a meeting, trying a new activity, or reaching out to someone you admire.
2. **Set Realistic Expectations:** Don't expect to be fearless overnight. Building courage takes time and practice. Be patient with yourself and celebrate each small victory along the way.
3. **Challenge Negative Self-Talk:** When those self-doubting thoughts creep in, counter them with positive affirmations. Remind yourself of your strengths, your accomplishments, and your potential.
4. **Visualize Success:** Before facing a fear, take a few moments to visualize yourself succeeding. See yourself feeling confident, capable, and in control.
5. **Find a Support System:** Surround yourself with people who believe in you and encourage you to step outside your comfort zone. Having a support system can make a huge difference when facing your fears.

Remember: Building courage is a process, not an event. It's about taking small, consistent steps towards your fears, learning from your experiences, and celebrating your progress along the way. So start flexing those courage muscles today, and watch your confidence, resilience, and overall well-being soar.

EXERCISE: FEAR LADDER

Alright, my friend, let's get practical. It's time to face those fears head-on. But don't worry, we're not going to throw you into the deep end right away. Instead, we're going to take a gradual approach, one step at a time. Think of it like climbing a ladder, starting with the easiest rung and working your way up to the top. This is your Fear Ladder.

WHY A FEAR LADDER?

The Fear Ladder is a powerful tool for overcoming anxieties and phobias. It works by gradually exposing you to your fears in a controlled and manageable way. This exposure helps to desensitize you to your fears, reducing their intensity and power over time. It's like dipping your toe in the water before diving in headfirst – it allows you to build up your courage and confidence step by step.

BUILDING YOUR FEAR LADDER

1. **Identify Your Fears:** Take a look at the "What If" Inventory you created on Day 1. Select one fear that you'd like to work on. It could be a fear of public speaking, a fear of rejection, or any other fear that's been holding you back.
2. **Break Down Your Fear:** Divide your chosen fear into smaller, more manageable steps. For example, if your fear is public speaking, your steps might look like this:
    - Step 1: Practice speaking in front of a mirror.

- Step 2: Talk to a trusted friend or family member.
- Step 3: Speak in front of a small group of friends.
- Step 4: Join a public speaking group or class.
- Step 5: Give a presentation to a larger audience.

3. **Rate Your Fear:** Assign a fear rating to each step on your ladder, using a scale of 1 to 10 (1 being the least scary, 10 being the most scary). This will help you gauge your progress and track your success.
4. **Start Climbing:** Begin with the easiest step on your ladder. Practice this step repeatedly until your fear rating decreases significantly. Once you feel comfortable, move on to the next step.

TIPS FOR CLIMBING YOUR FEAR LADDER

- **Take it Slow:** Don't rush the process. Allow yourself plenty of time to feel comfortable at each step before moving on to the next.
- **Celebrate Your Successes:** Acknowledge and celebrate each step you overcome. This will boost your confidence and motivation to keep going.
- **Be Kind to Yourself:** Don't beat yourself up if you have setbacks or if your progress is slower than you'd like. Remember, this is a journey, not a race.
- **Seek Support:** If you're struggling, don't hesitate to reach out to a trusted friend, family member, therapist, or coach for support.

THE REWARDS OF CLIMBING

As you climb your Fear Ladder, you'll start to notice a remarkable shift. Your fears will gradually lose their grip on you. You'll gain confidence, resilience, and a renewed sense of empowerment. You'll start to see challenges as opportunities for growth, rather than obstacles to avoid.

Most importantly, you'll open yourself up to new possibilities and experiences that were once out of reach. You'll be able to

pursue your dreams, take risks, and live a life that's truly authentic and fulfilling.

Remember, the Fear Ladder is not just about overcoming a specific fear. It's about developing a mindset of courage and resilience that you can apply to any challenge life throws your way. So embrace the process, celebrate your victories, and keep climbing towards a life of "no more what ifs."

Your Next Step

Now it's your turn to create your own Fear Ladder. Take some time to reflect on your fears and identify one that you're ready to tackle. Break it down into manageable steps, rate your fear levels, and start climbing. Remember, every step you take is a step towards freedom, empowerment, and a life lived without regrets.

Your journey to "no more what ifs" begins now.

Day 6: Letting Go of Regret

Think of regret as a heavy backpack you've been carrying around for years. It's filled with the weight of past mistakes, missed opportunities, and "should haves." This backpack slows you down, drains your energy, and prevents you from moving forward with confidence.

Today, we're going to unpack that backpack.

It's time to let go of the regrets that have been holding you hostage. It's time to forgive yourself, learn from the past, and embrace a future free from the chains of what might have been.

THE BURDEN OF REGRET

Regret is a complex emotion that can manifest in many ways. It can be a gnawing feeling in the pit of your stomach, a persistent thought that won't go away, or a deep sadness for what could have been. It can affect our relationships, our careers, our health, and our overall well-being.

But why do we hold onto regret? Often, it's because we

believe that by dwelling on our past mistakes, we can somehow change them or prevent them from happening again. We may feel that

we deserve to suffer for our perceived shortcomings, or that our regrets serve as a constant reminder to never make those mistakes again.

However, the truth is that regret rarely serves us in a positive way. It keeps us stuck in the past, robs us of our present joy, and clouds our vision for the future. It's like trying to drive a car while constantly looking in the rearview mirror - you're bound to crash.

THE FREEDOM OF FORGIVENESS

The first step in letting go of regret is forgiveness. This means forgiving yourself for any past mistakes or perceived shortcomings. It also means forgiving others who may have hurt you or contributed to your feelings of regret.

Forgiveness doesn't mean condoning the behavior or forgetting what happened. It simply means choosing to release the anger, resentment, and pain that are holding you back. It's a decision to move forward with grace and understanding, both for yourself and for others.

LEARNING FROM THE PAST

Regret can be a powerful teacher if we allow it to be. Instead of dwelling on what went wrong, ask yourself, "What can I learn from this experience?" Identify the lessons you've learned and how you can apply them to your future choices.

Remember, mistakes are not failures. They are opportunities for growth and transformation. Embrace your past experiences,

both the good and the bad, as valuable stepping stones on your journey.

CREATING A REGRET-FREE FUTURE

Letting go of regret is not a one-time event; it's an ongoing process. It requires a commitment to self-compassion, forgiveness, and a willingness to learn from your past. But the rewards are immense. When you release the burden of regret, you free yourself to live a life of purpose, passion, and joy.

In the following sections, we'll explore practical techniques for forgiving yourself and others, learning from your past, and creating a future that you'll look back on with pride and satisfaction.

FORGIVENESS: THE KEY TO FREEDOM

Imagine carrying around a backpack filled with heavy stones. Each stone represents a regret, a past mistake, a hurt you've experienced. With every step you take, the weight of the backpack pulls you down, making it harder to move forward, to breathe freely, to simply *be*.

That's what holding onto regret feels like. It's a heavy burden that weighs on our hearts, minds, and even our bodies. It can manifest as guilt, shame, anger, and resentment – emotions that sap our energy, drain our joy, and keep us stuck in the past.

But what if you could lay down that backpack? What if you could release those stones and walk free from the weight of regret? That's where forgiveness comes in.

THE POWER OF FORGIVENESS

Forgiveness is not about condoning or excusing hurtful actions. It's about acknowledging the pain that was caused and making a conscious decision to release the negative emotions associated with it. It's about recognizing that holding onto anger and resentment only hurts us in the long run.

When we forgive, we don't forget what happened, but we choose to let go of the emotional baggage that keeps us tied to the past. We create space for healing, growth, and new beginnings.

SELF-FORGIVENESS: THE FIRST STEP

Often, the hardest person to forgive is ourselves. We tend to be our own harshest critics, replaying our mistakes and berating ourselves for our shortcomings. But self-forgiveness is essential for inner peace and moving forward.

It's important to remember that we are all human. We all make mistakes. We all have moments where we fall short of our own expectations. It's part of the human experience.

Forgiving ourselves doesn't mean condoning our mistakes or pretending they didn't happen. It means acknowledging our humanity, accepting that we're not perfect, and giving ourselves permission to learn and grow from our experiences.

FORGIVING OTHERS: A PATH TO PEACE

Forgiving others can be even more challenging than forgiving ourselves. When someone has hurt us deeply, it can be difficult
to let go of the anger and resentment. But holding onto those emotions only keeps us trapped in the cycle of pain.

Forgiveness is not about forgetting or condoning the other person's actions. It's about freeing ourselves from the negative emotions that hold us captive. It's about recognizing that we deserve peace and happiness, regardless of what others have done to us.

Forgiveness is a gift we give ourselves. It allows us to move forward with a lighter heart, a clearer mind, and a renewed sense of purpose.

THE FREEDOM OF FORGIVENESS

When we forgive, we unlock a powerful force within ourselves – the power to heal, to grow, and to create a life that we truly love. Forgiveness allows us to:

- **Let Go of the Past:** By releasing the emotional baggage of regret, we free ourselves from the past and create space for new possibilities.
- **Heal from Emotional Wounds:** Forgiveness allows us to process the pain and move towards healing and emotional well-being.
- **Improve Relationships:** Forgiving others can mend broken relationships and create deeper connections.

- **Reduce Stress and Anxiety:** Holding onto anger and resentment can take a toll on our mental and physical health. Forgiveness releases this tension and promotes inner peace.
- **Find Inner Peace:** Forgiveness is not about the other person; it's about finding peace within ourselves. It allows us to move forward with a lighter heart and a clearer mind.

Forgiveness is a choice. It's not always easy, but it's always worth it. When we choose to forgive, we liberate ourselves from the shackles of regret and open ourselves up to a life of freedom, joy, and purpose.

Remember: Forgiveness is not a one-time event; it's a process that takes time, patience, and self-compassion. Be kind to yourself as you navigate this journey. Seek support from loved ones, therapists, or spiritual advisors if needed. The path to forgiveness may not be easy, but the rewards are immeasurable.

LEARNING FROM THE PAST

Regret, while often painful, doesn't have to be a life sentence. It can be a powerful teacher, guiding us towards growth, wisdom, and better choices in the future. Let's shift our perspective and explore how we can transform regret into a valuable asset on our journey to a regret-free life.

REGRET AS A REARVIEW MIRROR

Think of regret as a rearview mirror in your car. It allows you to glance back at the road you've traveled, but it's not meant to be your primary focus. While it's important to acknowledge and learn from past mistakes, constantly staring in the rearview mirror can prevent you from seeing the road ahead and enjoying the scenery.

Similarly, dwelling on past regrets can keep you stuck in a cycle of negativity and self-blame. It can cloud your judgment, stifle your creativity, and prevent you from taking action towards your goals. However, if you use regret as a tool for reflection and learning, it can become a catalyst for positive change.

IDENTIFYING LESSONS LEARNED

Every experience, even the ones we regret, offers valuable lessons. By reflecting on your past regrets, you can gain insights into your values, your decision-making patterns, and the areas where you need to grow.

Here are some questions to help you identify the lessons hidden within your regrets:

- *What was the situation that led to this regret?*
- *What were the choices I made, and why did I make them?*
- *What were the consequences of those choices?*
- *What would I do differently if I could go back in time?*
- *What have I learned about myself and my values through this experience?*

Take some time to reflect on your past regrets and answer these questions honestly. You may be surprised at the wisdom and insights that emerge.

APPLYING LESSONS TO FUTURE CHOICES

Once you've identified the lessons from your past regrets, the next step is to apply them to your future choices. This is where regret transforms into wisdom.

Here are some practical ways to apply the lessons you've learned:

1. **Make Amends:** If your regret involves hurting someone else, apologize and take steps to repair the relationship.
2. **Change Your Behavior:** If your regret stems from a pattern of behavior, commit to making positive changes. Seek support from a therapist, coach, or trusted friend if needed.
3. **Set New Boundaries:** If your regret involves overextending yourself or neglecting your own needs, establish healthy boundaries to protect your time, energy, and well-being.
4. **Make Different Choices:** When faced with similar situations in the future, use the lessons you've learned to make more informed and aligned choices.
5. **Practice Self-Forgiveness:** Forgive yourself for past mistakes and release the burden of regret. Remember, you're human, and everyone makes mistakes.

THE GIFT OF HINDSIGHT

As the saying goes, "Hindsight is 20/20." With the benefit of hindsight, we can often see our past choices more clearly and understand why we made them. This doesn't mean we should dwell on our mistakes, but it does mean we can use them as opportunities for growth and transformation.

Remember, regret is not a sign of weakness. It's a sign that you're human, that you care about making good choices, and that you're committed to learning and growing. By embracing regret as a teacher, you can transform your past experiences into valuable lessons that will guide you towards a more fulfilling, purposeful, and regret-free future.

EXERCISE: REGRET RELEASE RITUAL

Regret can feel like a heavy weight, dragging us down and preventing us from moving forward. It can be a persistent voice in our heads, reminding us of past mistakes, missed opportunities, or words left unspoken. But holding onto regret doesn't serve us; it keeps us trapped in the past, unable to fully embrace the present and create a brighter future.

It's time to release that weight, to let go of the regrets that are holding you back. It's time to reclaim your power and step into a life of freedom, purpose, and no more "what ifs."

THE REGRET RELEASE RITUALS

There are many ways to symbolically release regret. The most important thing is to choose a method that resonates with you and feels meaningful. Here are a few options to consider:

1. The Letter of Forgiveness:

- Write a letter to yourself or to someone else involved in the regret. Express your feelings honestly, acknowledging the hurt or pain caused.
- Forgive yourself or the other person for any perceived wrongs. Forgiveness doesn't mean condoning the action; it means freeing yourself from the emotional burden.
- Optionally, you can read the letter aloud, either to yourself or to a trusted friend or therapist.
- Destroy the letter in a way that feels symbolic, such as tearing it up, burning it, or burying it. As you do so, visualize the regret leaving your body and mind.

2. The Burning Ceremony:

- Write down your regrets on individual slips of paper.
- Gather in a safe place, such as a fireplace, bonfire, or even a candle flame.
- As you burn each slip of paper, repeat a releasing affirmation, such as "I release this regret. I forgive myself and others. I am free."
- Visualize the regret turning to smoke and ash, dissipating into the air and leaving you lighter and more at peace.

3. The Water Release:

- Write your regrets on biodegradable paper.
- Find a natural body of water, such as a river, lake, or ocean.
- As you gently place the paper in the water, say a prayer or affirmation of release.
- Watch as the water carries away your regrets, symbolizing a fresh start and a renewed sense of possibility.

4. The Releasing Ceremony:

- Create a personalized ceremony that feels meaningful to you.
- This could involve lighting candles, playing music, using crystals or other sacred objects, or incorporating elements of nature.
- Speak aloud your regrets, then release them through words, movement, or any other form of expression that feels right.
- Conclude your ceremony with a celebration of your newfound freedom.

ADDITIONAL TIPS FOR A POWERFUL RITUAL:

- Set the scene: Create a peaceful and sacred space for your ritual. This could be a quiet room in your home, a secluded spot in nature, or any other place where you feel safe and comfortable.
- Light a candle: Candles can create a calming and

reflective atmosphere. Choose a scent that you find soothing and relaxing.
- Play calming music: Soft music can help you relax and focus on the present moment.
- Use essential oils: Certain essential oils, such as lavender or frankincense, are known for their calming and healing properties.
- Connect with your body: Before and after the ritual, take a few deep breaths and focus on your body sensations. This can help you ground yourself and release any lingering tension.
- Write in your journal: After the ritual, take some time to journal about your experience. Reflect on how you feel and what insights you gained.

Remember, the most important element of any regret release ritual is the intention behind it. As you perform your chosen ritual, focus on letting go of the past, forgiving yourself and others, and embracing a future filled with possibility.

Your past does not define you. You are not your mistakes. You are capable of growth, healing, and transformation. By releasing your regrets, you open yourself up to a life of freedom, joy, and fulfillment. You reclaim your power and step into the person you were always meant to be.

Day 7: Gratitude Journal

Have you ever noticed how easy it is to get caught up in the negatives? To focus on what's going wrong, what we lack, or what we wish we could change? It's like our brains are wired to hone in on the problems, the challenges, and the things that aren't quite right in our lives.

But what if I told you there's a simple yet powerful tool that can help you shift your focus, boost your mood, and even improve your overall well-being? It's not a magic pill or a complex formula; it's as simple as keeping a gratitude journal.

Gratitude journaling is the practice of regularly writing down things you're thankful for. It can be as simple as jotting down three things you appreciate each day or as elaborate as writing detailed reflections on your blessings. Regardless of the format, the act of focusing on gratitude has a profound impact on our minds and bodies.

THE SCIENCE OF GRATITUDE

Research has shown that gratitude is more than just a nice

feeling; it's a powerful emotion with tangible benefits. Studies have linked gratitude to:

- **Increased Happiness:** Gratitude helps us savor positive experiences, feel more joy, and appreciate the good things in life.
- **Reduced Stress:** Focusing on gratitude can lower cortisol levels (the stress hormone) and promote relaxation.
- **Improved Relationships:** Expressing gratitude to others strengthens our social bonds and deepens our connections.
- **Better Sleep:** Gratitude journaling before bed can help calm the mind and promote restful sleep.
- **Increased Resilience:** Grateful individuals tend to be more optimistic, adaptable, and better equipped to handle adversity.

These are just a few of the many benefits that gratitude can bring into your life. And the best part is, it's a skill you can develop with practice.

GRATITUDE: A DAILY PRACTICE

Think of gratitude as a muscle that you can strengthen with exercise. The more you practice gratitude, the more naturally it will become a part of your mindset.

Here are a few simple ways to incorporate gratitude into your daily routine:

- **Start a Gratitude Journal:** Dedicate a few minutes each day to write down 3-5 things you're grateful for.
- **Express Gratitude to Others:** Tell your loved ones how much you appreciate them. Write a thank-you note or simply offer a sincere compliment.
- **Savor Positive Experiences:** Take the time to fully enjoy the good moments in your life, whether it's a delicious meal, a beautiful sunset, or a joyful conversation.
- **Notice the Little Things:** Appreciate the small things that often go unnoticed, like a warm cup of coffee, a comfortable bed, or a kind gesture from a stranger.

YOUR GRATITUDE JOURNEY BEGINS TODAY

Today marks the beginning of your gratitude journey. In this chapter, you'll dive deeper into the science of gratitude, explore different ways to practice it, and start your own gratitude journal.

Remember, gratitude is a gift you give yourself. It's a simple yet profound way to cultivate happiness, resilience, and a deeper appreciation for life's blessings. So grab a pen and paper, open your heart, and let's get started.

THE SCIENCE OF GRATITUDE

Gratitude might sound like a fluffy, feel-good concept, but don't be fooled. It's a powerful tool backed by science that can literally rewire your brain for happiness, resilience, and well-being.

Think of gratitude as a muscle. The more you use it, the

stronger it gets. And just like physical exercise, practicing gratitude yields incredible benefits for both your mind and body.

THE HAPPINESS BOOST

Ever notice how focusing on what you don't have can quickly spiral into a downward mood? Gratitude works in the opposite direction. When you actively seek out things to be thankful for, your brain releases dopamine and serotonin, those feel-good neurotransmitters that lift your spirits and create a sense of joy.

This isn't just a fleeting feeling, either. Studies have shown that people who regularly practice gratitude experience a lasting increase in happiness and overall life satisfaction. They tend to be more optimistic, enthusiastic, and energetic. Who wouldn't want that?

THE STRESS BUSTER

Stress is a fact of life, but gratitude can be its kryptonite. When you're feeling overwhelmed or anxious, taking a moment to focus on what you're grateful for can shift your perspective and calm your nervous system.

Research shows that grateful people tend to have lower levels of cortisol, the stress hormone. They're also better at managing stress and bouncing back from adversity. Gratitude acts like a buffer, helping you navigate life's challenges with greater ease and resilience.

THE RELATIONSHIP BUILDER

Gratitude isn't just about feeling good on the inside; it can also transform your relationships. When you express appreciation to others, it not only makes them feel valued and loved but also strengthens your bond with them.

Think about it: When was the last time someone genuinely thanked you for something you did? How did it make you feel? Chances are, it made you feel seen, appreciated, and more connected to that person.

Gratitude is a two-way street. When you make it a habit to express gratitude to your loved ones, friends, colleagues, and even strangers, you create a ripple effect of positivity. You foster an environment of appreciation, kindness, and connection, which benefits everyone involved.

SHIFTING YOUR FOCUS

One of the most powerful aspects of gratitude is its ability to shift our focus from what we lack to what we have. It's so easy to get caught up in the comparison game, constantly feeling like we're not enough or don't have enough. But gratitude helps us break free from this trap.

When you start focusing on the good in your life – your health, your loved ones, your unique talents, the simple pleasures that bring you joy – you realize how much you actually have to be thankful for. It's a subtle shift in perspective, but it can have a profound impact on your overall happiness and well-being.

So, How Do You Practice Gratitude?

The great thing about gratitude is that it's not complicated. There are many simple ways to incorporate it into your daily life:

- **Keep a gratitude journal:** Write down 3-5 things you're grateful for each day.
- **Express appreciation to others:** Say "thank you" more often, write thank-you notes, or express your gratitude in person.
- **Savor positive experiences:** Take the time to fully enjoy the good moments in your life.
- **Notice the little things:** Pay attention to the small details that often go unnoticed, like a beautiful sunset, a delicious meal, or a kind gesture.
- **Practice mindfulness:** Pay attention to the present moment and appreciate the simple joys of life.

Remember, gratitude is a skill that takes practice. But the more you make it a habit, the more natural it will become. And the benefits? Well, they're simply too good to ignore.

A DAILY PRACTICE

So, you've dipped your toes into the gratitude pool, and maybe you've even felt a ripple of its warmth and positivity. But how do you turn gratitude from a fleeting feeling into a daily practice, a way of life? Let's dive into the practical steps that can make gratitude your superpower.

THE GRATITUDE JOURNAL: YOUR DAILY GRATITUDE WORKOUT

Think of your gratitude journal as a workout for your happiness muscle. Just like lifting weights strengthens your body, writing down what you're grateful for each day strengthens your mind's ability to focus on the positive. But don't worry, this workout doesn't require fancy equipment or a gym membership – just a pen, a notebook, and a few minutes of your time.

Start simple. Each day, jot down three things you're grateful for. These can be big things like your health, family, or a fulfilling career, or they can be small things like the taste of your morning coffee, a sunny day, or a friendly smile from a stranger. There's no right or wrong way to do it. The key is to make it a habit.

Here are some tips to make the most of your gratitude journal:

- **Be Specific:** Instead of just writing "my family," try something like, "I'm grateful for my sister's contagious laugh and the way she always makes me feel loved." The more specific you are, the more vividly you'll experience the feeling of gratitude.
- **Go Beyond the Obvious:** It's easy to be grateful for the good things in life. But what about the challenges? Can you find something to be grateful for even in the midst of a difficult situation? This can be a powerful way to reframe your perspective and find strength in adversity.

- **Make it a Ritual:** Choose a time of day that works for you, whether it's first thing in the morning, during your lunch break, or before bed. Make it a consistent ritual so that gratitude becomes a natural part of your daily routine.

GRATITUDE ON THE GO: FINDING THANKFULNESS IN EVERY MOMENT

Your gratitude practice doesn't have to be confined to your journal. You can infuse gratitude into your daily life in countless ways. Here are a few ideas:

- **Express Your Appreciation:** Make a habit of saying "thank you" to the people in your life who make a difference. Whether it's your partner, your kids, your barista, or your mail carrier, let them know that you appreciate them.
- **Savor the Moment:** Take a moment each day to fully experience something you're grateful for. It could be the warmth of the sun on your skin, the taste of your favorite food, or the sound of laughter. Slow down and savor the experience.
- **Practice Mindful Gratitude:** Throughout your day, pause and notice the little things that bring you joy. It could be a beautiful sunset, a kind gesture from a stranger, or the feeling of accomplishment after completing a task. Take a moment to acknowledge and appreciate these small moments of gratitude.

THE RIPPLE EFFECT OF GRATITUDE

As you cultivate a daily gratitude practice, you'll start to notice a shift in your perspective. The negative thoughts that once consumed your mind will begin to fade, replaced by a sense of appreciation and abundance. You'll find yourself feeling more positive, more resilient, and more connected to the world around you.

But the benefits of gratitude don't stop there. Gratitude is contagious. When you express your gratitude to others, it creates a ripple effect of positivity that can spread far and wide. By sharing your gratitude, you not only uplift others but also reinforce your own sense of appreciation.

So, are you ready to make gratitude your daily practice? Remember, it's not about being perfect or having a picture-perfect life. It's about finding the good in every moment, no matter how small. It's about shifting your focus from what you lack to what you have. And it's about embracing the power of gratitude to transform your life from the inside out.

EXERCISE: GRATITUDE JOURNAL

Okay, friend, grab your journal or a blank piece of paper. If you're a digital native, open up your favorite note-taking app. It's time for a gratitude download!

I know what you're thinking. "Another journal exercise?" Hear me out. This isn't just about filling pages with words; it's about rewiring your brain for positivity and joy. It's about noticing and appreciating the good stuff, even on the toughest days.

Remember, we're not chasing some elusive state of eternal bliss where nothing ever goes wrong. Life throws curveballs, that's a given. But a gratitude practice isn't about denying challenges; it's about finding those glimmers of light that exist even in the darkest corners.

Think of your gratitude journal as a treasure chest. Each day, you'll add a few gems to it—small moments, unexpected kindnesses, things that made you smile. Over time, this chest will overflow with precious reminders of the good in your life.

Your First Entry: Finding the Gold Nuggets

Think back over your day. What moments stand out? Did a stranger hold the door for you? Did you share a laugh with a friend? Did the sun feel warm on your skin?

Don't worry about finding profound epiphanies or earth-shattering events. Sometimes, the most ordinary moments hold the greatest magic. Did your coffee taste extra delicious this morning? Did you hear a song that lifted your spirits? Did you simply wake up feeling rested and energized?

Here's a tip: Be specific. Instead of writing, "I'm grateful for my family," try something like, "I'm grateful for the hilarious text my sister sent me today." Specificity brings depth and richness to your gratitude practice.

Putting Pen to Paper (or Fingers to Keyboard)

Now, let's get those thoughts down on paper (or screen). Start with the phrase "I am grateful for..." and then let your thoughts flow. Don't overthink it; just write from the heart.

Here are a few prompts to get you started:

- **Simple Pleasures:** I am grateful for the warm sunshine on my face this afternoon.

- **Acts of Kindness:** I am grateful for the stranger who helped me carry my groceries.
- **Moments of Joy:** I am grateful for the laughter I shared with my friend during our coffee date.
- **Personal Achievements:** I am grateful for the progress I made on my project today.
- **Unexpected Blessings:** I am grateful for the beautiful rainbow I saw after the storm.
- **Challenges Overcome:** I am grateful for the strength I found to face a difficult situation.

Remember, there are no right or wrong answers. Your gratitude journal is yours and yours alone. The most important thing is to be honest, specific, and to write from a place of genuine appreciation.

Why Three Things?

You might be wondering why I'm suggesting you start with three things to be grateful for. The number isn't magical, but it's a good starting point. It's enough to get your gratitude juices flowing without feeling overwhelming.

As you get into the habit of journaling, you can increase the number of things you write about each day. You might even find that your gratitude list spills over onto multiple pages!

THE RIPPLE EFFECT

Gratitude isn't just a feel-good exercise; it's a powerful tool for transformation. When you focus on the good in your life, you train your brain to see more of it. You start to notice the abundance that surrounds you, even in the midst of challenges.

Gratitude also has a ripple effect. When you express gratitude to others, it not only makes them feel good, but it also strengthens your bond with them. It creates a positive energy that radiates outward, uplifting everyone around you.

So, as you embark on this gratitude journey, remember:

- **Be consistent:** Aim to write in your journal every day, even if it's just a few sentences.
- **Be specific:** Focus on details and specific experiences rather than general statements.
- **Be open:** Allow yourself to feel the emotions that arise as you express gratitude.
- **Be curious:** Explore different ways of practicing gratitude, beyond just writing in your journal.

Now, take a deep breath, pick up your pen, and let the gratitude flow. Remember, this is your journey, your story, and your unique experience. Embrace it fully and allow gratitude to become a guiding force in your life.

Day 8: Self-Talk Audit

Ever catch yourself saying things like, "I'm not good enough," "I always mess things up," or "I'll never be able to do that"? If so, you're not alone. We all have an inner critic—a voice in our heads that whispers doubts, criticisms, and fears. This inner dialogue, often referred to as self-talk, can have a profound impact on our confidence, motivation, and overall well-being.

Negative self-talk is like a broken record, playing the same limiting beliefs on repeat. It can sabotage our efforts, undermine our confidence, and keep us stuck in the same patterns of fear and regret. It's the voice that says, "Don't even try," "You're going to fail," or "Why bother?"

But here's the good news: You're not powerless against your inner critic. You have the ability to rewrite your inner script, challenge those negative thoughts, and create a more empowering narrative. That's where the self-talk audit comes in.

Think of the self-talk audit as a detective mission to uncover the hidden messages your inner critic is sending you. It's a chance to become aware of the negative patterns that are holding you back and to start replacing them with more positive and affirming beliefs.

WHY A SELF-TALK AUDIT IS ESSENTIAL:

- **Awareness:** The first step to changing negative self-talk is becoming aware of it. The self-talk audit helps you identify the specific phrases, words, and tone of voice your inner critic uses.
- **Patterns:** By tracking your self-talk over time, you'll start to notice patterns. Are there certain situations or triggers that tend to evoke negative thoughts? This awareness is crucial for understanding the root causes of your inner critic.
- **Reframing:** Once you've identified your negative thoughts, you can start to challenge and reframe them. This involves replacing those limiting beliefs with more positive and empowering ones.
- **Empowerment:** By taking control of your inner dialogue, you reclaim your power. You shift from being a victim of your thoughts to becoming the author of your own story.

Over the next few days, we'll dive deeper into the self-talk audit process. You'll learn how to track your thoughts, identify patterns, and develop strategies for reframing negativity. By the end, you'll have a powerful toolkit for transforming your inner dialogue and creating a more positive, supportive, and empowering relationship with yourself.

So, let's get started on this transformative journey. It's time to silence that inner critic and embrace the powerful voice within you that's ready to rise.

BECOMING AWARE OF YOUR INNER CRITIC

Have you ever had a little voice inside your head that whispers doubts, criticisms, and negativity? That voice, my friend, is your inner critic. It's that nagging feeling that tells you you're not good enough, smart enough, or capable enough. It's the voice that replays your past mistakes, amplifies your insecurities, and feeds your fears.

Let's be honest, we all have an inner critic. It's a natural part of the human experience. But when that inner critic becomes overly critical and negative, it can wreak havoc on our self-esteem, confidence, and overall well-being.

THE SNEAKY WAYS OF YOUR INNER CRITIC

Your inner critic is a master of disguise. It can show up in various forms:

- **The Perfectionist:** This voice demands flawlessness and berates you for any perceived mistakes or shortcomings. It tells you that you're not good enough unless everything is perfect.
- **The Catastrophizer:** This voice magnifies the negative and expects the worst-case scenario. It tells you that you're doomed to fail and that any setback is a sign of impending doom.
- **The Comparer:** This voice constantly compares you to

others, making you feel inadequate and inferior. It tells you that everyone else is more successful, attractive, or talented than you.
- **The Blamer:** This voice blames you for everything that goes wrong, even if it's outside your control. It tells you that you're the reason for your failures and that you don't deserve good things.

These are just a few examples of how your inner critic can manifest. It's important to recognize your inner critic's voice and the specific messages it sends you.

THE DAMAGE DONE BY NEGATIVE SELF-TALK

Negative self-talk isn't just harmless chatter; it can have a profound impact on your life. It can:

- **Undermine Your Confidence:** When you constantly criticize yourself, it erodes your self-belief and makes it harder to trust your own judgment.
- **Fuel Fear and Regret:** Negative self-talk amplifies your fears and makes you more likely to dwell on past mistakes and missed opportunities.
- **Sabotage Your Success:** Your inner critic can hold you back from taking risks, pursuing your dreams, and achieving your goals.
- **Impact Your Mental Health:** Chronic negative self-talk can contribute to anxiety, depression, and other mental health issues.
- **Strain Your Relationships:** When you're constantly

criticizing yourself, it can be difficult to connect with others on a deeper level.

IDENTIFYING YOUR INNER CRITIC'S VOICE

The first step to overcoming your inner critic is to become aware of its presence. Start paying attention to your thoughts and notice when you're engaging in negative self-talk. What are the specific words and phrases you use? What situations or triggers tend to bring out your inner critic?

Here are some common negative thought patterns to look out for:

- **All-or-Nothing Thinking:** Seeing things in black and white terms, with no middle ground.
- **Overgeneralization:** Making sweeping negative conclusions based on one incident.
- **Mental Filtering:** Focusing only on the negative and ignoring the positive.
- **Personalization:** Blaming yourself for things that are outside of your control.

Once you become aware of your inner critic's voice and the specific messages it sends you, you can start to challenge those thoughts and replace them with more positive and empowering ones. This is where the practice of reframing comes in. We'll delve deeper into reframing in the next section, but for now, just start paying attention to your thoughts and notice when your inner critic is trying to take the wheel.

Remember, you have the power to change your inner

dialogue. By becoming aware of your negative self-talk and challenging its validity, you can start to cultivate a more positive and supportive inner voice.

THE POWER OF REFRAMING

Our minds are like a radio station, constantly broadcasting a stream of thoughts, beliefs, and interpretations. Some of these transmissions are upbeat and encouraging, while others are filled with static and negativity. The problem is, we often tune into the negative station without even realizing it. We get so caught up in the drama of our self-defeating thoughts that we forget we have the power to change the channel.

That's where the power of reframing comes in. Reframing is like taking a pair of mental scissors and cutting up that negative script, rearranging the words, and rewriting a new story. It's about challenging the validity of our negative thoughts and replacing them with more positive and empowering ones.

Let's face it, we all have an inner critic. That voice that tells us we're not good enough, smart enough, or capable enough. It's the voice that whispers doubt, amplifies our fears, and sabotages our dreams. But here's the secret: that inner critic is not the ultimate authority on who we are or what we can achieve. It's simply a thought pattern, a habit of thinking that we've developed over time.

And just like any habit, it can be changed.

HOW REFRAMING WORKS

Reframing is not about denying reality or pretending that

everything is perfect. It's about shifting our perspective, looking at situations from a different angle, and choosing a more empowering interpretation. It's about replacing those self-defeating thoughts with ones that uplift us, motivate us, and move us closer to our goals.

Here's a simple example:

Negative thought: "I'm such a failure. I'll never be successful."

Reframe: "I've faced challenges before, and I've learned from them. I'm capable of achieving my goals."

Notice how the reframe doesn't deny the existence of challenges or setbacks. It simply shifts the focus from defeatism to resilience and growth. It acknowledges the past while emphasizing the potential for a brighter future.

WHY REFRAMING MATTERS

Our thoughts have a powerful impact on our emotions, actions, and overall well-being. When we constantly bombard ourselves with negative thoughts, we create a self-fulfilling prophecy of failure and disappointment. But when we reframe those thoughts into positive ones, we set ourselves up for success and fulfillment.

Reframing can help us:

- **Reduce stress and anxiety:** Negative thoughts often trigger stress and anxiety. By reframing those thoughts, we can calm our minds and bodies, creating a sense of peace and well-being.
- **Increase self-confidence:** When we believe in ourselves

and our abilities, we're more likely to take risks and pursue our dreams. Reframing can help us build that self-belief.
- **Improve relationships:** Negative thoughts about ourselves can also impact our relationships. By reframing those thoughts, we can show up as more confident, positive, and loving partners, friends, and family members.
- **Overcome obstacles:** When faced with challenges, our thoughts can either empower us or hold us back. By reframing negative thoughts, we can find the strength and resilience to persevere.

PRACTICAL TIPS FOR REFRAMING

Here are some practical tips for reframing negative thoughts:

1. **Identify the thought:** The first step is to become aware of your negative thoughts. Notice when they arise and what triggers them.
2. **Challenge its validity:** Ask yourself if the thought is true. Is there another way to look at the situation? What evidence do you have to support or refute this thought?
3. **Replace it with a positive alternative:** Come up with a more empowering thought that counters the negative one. Make sure the new thought is realistic and believable.
4. **Repeat, repeat, repeat:** Reframing takes practice. The

more you do it, the easier it will become. Eventually, positive thoughts will become your default setting.

Remember, you are not your thoughts. You have the power to choose which thoughts you focus on and which ones you let go of. By practicing the art of reframing, you can rewrite your inner dialogue, cultivate a more positive outlook.

EXERCISE: SELF-TALK AUDIT

Time to put on your detective hat and dive deeper into the world of your inner dialogue. Remember that pesky inner critic we talked about? The one who whispers doubts, anxieties, and limiting beliefs? It's time to expose their sneaky tactics and rewrite the script they've been feeding you.

WHY AUDIT YOUR SELF-TALK?

Think of your self-talk as a constant stream of commentary running in the background of your mind. It's like having a personal radio station that's either playing uplifting tunes or broadcasting a negativity marathon. The problem is, we often don't even realize what's playing until we tune in and listen closely.

This self-talk audit is your chance to become aware of the messages you're unconsciously sending yourself. By identifying negative patterns, you can challenge their validity, reframe them, and ultimately create a more empowering inner narrative.

HOW TO CONDUCT THE AUDIT

1. **Carry a Notebook (or Use Your Phone):** Keep a notebook handy or use a note-taking app on your phone. The key is to have a way to jot down your thoughts quickly and easily throughout the day.
2. **Tune In:** Pay attention to the thoughts that pop up in your mind, especially when you're feeling stressed, anxious, or discouraged. What are you saying to yourself? Are you focusing on your shortcomings, worrying about the future, or dwelling on past mistakes?
3. **Write it Down:** As soon as you notice a negative thought, write it down verbatim. Don't judge yourself or try to change it; simply record it as accurately as possible.
4. **Look for Patterns:** At the end of the day, review your notes. Do you notice any recurring themes or patterns? Are there certain situations that trigger negative self-talk? Recognizing these patterns is the first step towards changing them.
5. **Challenge the Validity:** For each negative thought, ask yourself: Is this really true? Is there another way to look at this situation? Are you being too hard on yourself?
6. **Reframe the Thought:** Rewrite the negative thought into a more positive and empowering statement. For example, instead of "I'm not good enough," try "I am capable and worthy." Instead of "I always mess things up," try "I learn from my mistakes and grow stronger."

Examples of Negative Self-Talk and Positive Reframes

Negative Self-Talk	Positive Reframe
"I'll never be able to achieve my goals."	"I am capable of achieving anything I set my mind to."
"I'm not smart enough for this."	"I am intelligent and capable of learning new things."
"I always make mistakes."	"I am human, and mistakes are opportunities for growth."
"I'm not worthy of love and happiness."	"I am deserving of love, joy, and all good things in life."
"I can't handle this challenge."	"I am resilient and can overcome any obstacle."

TIPS FOR SUCCESS

- **Be Honest:** Don't sugarcoat your thoughts. The more honest you are with yourself, the more effective this exercise will be.
- **Be Patient:** Changing your self-talk takes time and practice. Don't get discouraged if you don't see immediate results.
- **Be Kind to Yourself:** Speak to yourself with the same compassion and understanding you would offer a friend.
- **Celebrate Your Wins:** Every time you successfully reframe a negative thought, celebrate it! This positive reinforcement will help solidify the new, empowering message.

GOING BEYOND THE AUDIT

This self-talk audit is just the beginning. Once you've identified your negative patterns, you can start to actively challenge and reframe them in real-time. Whenever you catch yourself engaging in negative self-talk, pause, take a deep breath, and replace it with a positive affirmation.

Remember, your thoughts have power. By choosing to focus on empowering and uplifting messages, you can transform your inner dialogue and create a reality that reflects your true potential.

Day 9: Mindfulness Meditation

Ever feel like your mind is a runaway train, chugging along at breakneck speed with no brakes? Thoughts racing, worries piling up, "what ifs" echoing in your ears? It's exhausting, isn't it?

Today, we're going to introduce a powerful tool that can help you regain control of that train and find a sense of calm amidst the chaos. It's called mindfulness meditation.

Now, before you roll your eyes and think, "Oh great, another woo-woo concept," hear me out. Mindfulness isn't about chanting mantras or sitting cross-legged for hours on end (unless you want to, of course!). It's simply about paying attention to the present moment without judgment.

Think of it like this: your mind is a muscle, and just like any muscle, it needs training to become stronger and more flexible. Mindfulness meditation is like a workout for your mind, helping you build the mental strength and resilience to handle life's challenges with more grace and ease.

WHY MINDFULNESS MATTERS

So, why should you care about mindfulness? Well, research has
shown that it can have a profound impact on your mental and physical well-being. It can reduce stress, anxiety, and depression, improve focus and concentration, enhance creativity, and even boost your immune system.

But beyond the scientific benefits, mindfulness is a powerful tool for overcoming fear and regret. When we're caught up in the "what ifs" of the past or the anxieties of the future, we miss out on the beauty and richness of the present moment. Mindfulness brings us back to the here and now, where we can fully experience life as it unfolds.

It helps us break free from the cycle of rumination and worry, allowing us to see our thoughts and feelings with greater clarity and perspective. It teaches us to respond to challenges with more compassion and understanding, rather than reacting impulsively or getting caught up in negative emotions.

MINDFULNESS: NOT A QUICK FIX, BUT A POWERFUL PRACTICE

Now, let's be realistic: mindfulness isn't a magic pill that will instantly solve all your problems. It's a practice, something you need to cultivate over time. But even a few minutes of mindfulness each day can make a significant difference in your overall well-being and ability to navigate life's challenges.

Think of it as a daily investment in your mental health,

like brushing your teeth or eating a healthy meal. It's a simple yet powerful way to take care of yourself and build the inner strength you need to face whatever life throws your way.

In this chapter, we'll guide you through a simple mindfulness meditation exercise that you can easily incorporate into your

daily routine. We'll also discuss other ways to cultivate mindfulness in your everyday life, from mindful eating to mindful walking.

So, are you ready to give your mind a workout and discover the power of mindfulness for yourself? Let's dive in!

MINDFULNESS EXPLAINED

In our fast-paced, technology-driven world, it's easy to get swept away in the current of thoughts, worries, and endless to-do lists. Our minds often resemble a bustling marketplace, filled with noise and distractions that pull us away from the present moment. This constant mental chatter can lead to stress, anxiety, and rumination – that relentless replaying of negative thoughts and experiences.

But what if there was a way to quiet the noise, find inner peace, and reclaim control of your thoughts? Enter mindfulness.

WHAT IS MINDFULNESS?

Mindfulness is a simple yet powerful practice that involves paying full attention to the present moment without judgment. It's about being aware of your thoughts, emotions, bodily sensations, and the world around you – without getting caught up in them. It's like pressing the pause button on your mental chatter and tuning into the here and now.

Think of mindfulness as a muscle that you can strengthen with practice. Just as you would exercise your body to build strength and flexibility, you can train your mind to be more present, focused, and resilient.

THE BENEFITS OF MINDFULNESS

Research has shown that practicing mindfulness can have a profound impact on our well-being:

- **Stress Reduction:** Mindfulness helps us become aware of the physical and emotional signs of stress, allowing us to respond more effectively instead of reacting impulsively.
- **Anxiety Management:** By anchoring us in the present moment, mindfulness helps us break free from the cycle of worry and rumination that fuels anxiety.
- **Improved Focus and Concentration:** Regular mindfulness practice can enhance our ability to concentrate, stay on task, and be more productive.
- **Emotional Regulation:** Mindfulness allows us to observe our emotions without judgment, helping us manage difficult feelings and make more conscious choices.
- **Enhanced Self-Awareness:** Through mindfulness, we become more attuned to our thoughts, feelings, and bodily sensations, gaining valuable insights into ourselves.

HOW DOES MINDFULNESS WORK?

Mindfulness works by training our attention and cultivating a non-judgmental attitude towards our experiences. When we practice mindfulness, we learn to observe our thoughts and feelings as they arise, without getting caught up in them. This allows us to create a healthy distance between ourselves and our thoughts, reducing their power over us.

Imagine your thoughts as passing clouds in the sky. You can observe them, acknowledge them, and then let them drift away without getting entangled in their drama. This is the essence of mindfulness.

MINDFULNESS AND RUMINATION

Rumination is a common pattern of thinking where we dwell on negative thoughts and experiences, often leading to feelings of anxiety, depression, and helplessness. It's like a broken record that keeps playing the same track over and over again.

Mindfulness helps us break free from this cycle of rumination. By training our attention to the present moment, we can interrupt the negative thought patterns and create space for new, more positive perspectives. We learn to observe our thoughts without judgment, which reduces their intensity and allows us to choose how we respond to them.

Think of it like this: when we're caught up in rumination, we're driving a car with the rearview mirror firmly in our sight. We're constantly looking back at the past, reliving old hurts and mistakes. Mindfulness helps us turn our attention to the windshield, focusing on the present moment and the road ahead.

BRINGING MINDFULNESS INTO YOUR LIFE

Mindfulness can be practiced in many ways, from formal meditation to informal practices like mindful eating, walking, or even washing dishes. The key is to find practices that resonate with you and fit into your daily life.

Here are a few simple ways to incorporate mindfulness into your routine:

- **Start Small:** Even a few minutes of mindful breathing each day can make a difference.
- **Set Reminders:** Use phone alarms or sticky notes to remind yourself to pause and be present throughout the day.
- **Find a Quiet Space:** Create a peaceful environment where you can practice mindfulness without distractions.
- **Be Kind to Yourself:** Don't judge yourself if your mind wanders – it's natural. Simply bring your attention back to the present moment with kindness and compassion.
- **Explore Different Practices:** Experiment with different mindfulness techniques to find what works best for you.

Mindfulness is not a quick fix, but a lifelong journey of self-discovery and growth. By cultivating a non-judgmental awareness of the present moment, we can reduce stress, manage anxiety, overcome rumination, and live a more fulfilling and joyful life. So take a deep breath, let go of the past and the future, and embrace the power of the present moment.

A SIMPLE PRACTICE

Ready to dive into the world of mindfulness meditation? Don't worry, you don't need to be a Zen master or sit in a lotus pose to reap its benefits. In fact, you can practice mindfulness anytime, anywhere, even while you're washing dishes or waiting in line.

Mindfulness is simply the practice of paying full attention to the present moment without judgment. It's about noticing your thoughts, feelings, and bodily sensations without getting caught up in them. Think of it like being a curious observer of your own experience, rather than a judge.

Let's try a simple mindfulness meditation exercise together:

Finding Your Center

1. **Get Comfortable:** Find a quiet spot where you won't be disturbed. You can sit in a chair with your feet flat on the floor, or lie down if that's more comfortable. If you're sitting, keep your spine straight but not rigid.
2. **Close Your Eyes (or Soften Your Gaze):** Gently close your eyes, or if you prefer, soften your gaze and focus on a point in front of you.
3. **Bring Your Attention to Your Breath:** Notice the natural flow of your breath as it enters and leaves your

nostrils. Feel the rise and fall of your chest or abdomen. There's no need to control your breath; simply observe it.

4. **Anchor Yourself to the Present:** If your mind starts to wander (and it will!), gently bring your attention back to your breath. You can silently say to yourself, "Breathing in, I know I am breathing in. Breathing out, I know I am breathing out."
5. **Notice Sensations:** As you focus on your breath, also notice any sensations in your body. Do you feel tension in your shoulders? Tingling in your fingers? Warmth or coolness on your skin? Just observe these sensations without trying to change them.
6. **Welcome Your Thoughts and Feelings:** Thoughts and feelings will inevitably arise during meditation. Don't fight them or judge them. Simply acknowledge them and let them go, like clouds passing through the sky. You can say to yourself, "Thinking, thinking," or "Feeling, feeling."
7. **Be Kind to Yourself:** If you find yourself getting distracted or frustrated, don't worry. It's completely normal for the mind to wander. Just gently bring your attention back to your breath or body sensations. Remember, this is a practice, not a performance.
8. **Open Your Eyes (or Lift Your Gaze):** After a few minutes (you can start with 5 minutes and gradually increase), gently open your eyes or lift your gaze. Notice how you feel. Do you feel more relaxed? More centered? More present?

TIPS FOR MINDFUL LIVING

You can apply mindfulness not only during formal meditation but throughout your daily life:

- **Mindful Eating:** Pay attention to the taste, texture, and aroma of your food. Notice how your body feels as you eat.
- **Mindful Walking:** Focus on the sensations of your feet hitting the ground, the movement of your legs, and the feeling of the air on your skin.
- **Mindful Chores:** Bring your full attention to whatever task you're doing, whether it's washing dishes, folding laundry, or brushing your teeth.
- **Mindful Conversation:** Truly listen to the person you're talking to, without interrupting or planning your response. Notice their facial expressions, body language, and tone of voice.

Remember:

- **Consistency is Key:** Aim to practice mindfulness meditation daily, even if it's just for a few minutes.
- **Be Patient:** Mindfulness takes time and practice to cultivate. Don't get discouraged if your mind wanders. Simply bring your attention back to the present moment.
- **Be Kind to Yourself:** If you find yourself judging or criticizing your thoughts or feelings, gently remind yourself to be kind and compassionate.

- **Acceptance:** Accept whatever arises in your experience without judgment. This is the essence of mindfulness.

THE BENEFITS OF MINDFULNESS

The benefits of regular mindfulness practice are numerous and well-documented. Mindfulness can help you:

- **Reduce stress and anxiety:** By focusing on the present moment, you can let go of worries about the future and regrets about the past.
- **Improve focus and concentration:** Mindfulness trains your mind to stay present and attentive to the task at hand.
- **Cultivate self-awareness:** By observing your thoughts and feelings without judgment, you can gain a deeper understanding of yourself and your patterns.
- **Enhance emotional regulation:** Mindfulness helps you become more aware of your emotions and develop healthy ways of coping with them.
- **Improve relationships:** Mindfulness can help you become a more present and compassionate listener, leading to stronger and more meaningful connections with others.

By incorporating mindfulness into your life, you can create a calmer, more centered, and more joyful experience. You can tap into your inner wisdom, make wiser choices, and live a life that's aligned with your deepest values and aspirations.

EXERCISE: MINDFULNESS MEDITATION

Ready to take a break from the hustle and bustle of daily life? It's time for our mindfulness meditation exercise. Don't worry if you've never meditated before – I'll guide you through it step by step. And remember, mindfulness is like any skill; it takes practice and patience to master.

Setting the Stage:

1. **Find a Quiet Space:** Choose a place where you won't be disturbed for the next 5-10 minutes. It could be your bedroom, a cozy corner, or even a park bench.
2. **Get Comfortable:** Sit in a chair with your feet flat on the floor, or sit cross-legged on a cushion. You can also lie down if that's more comfortable. The key is to keep your spine straight but not rigid.
3. **Set a Timer:** Use your phone or a timer to track your meditation session. Start with 5 minutes and gradually increase the duration as you get more comfortable.

The Guided Meditation:

1. **Gently Close Your Eyes:** Or, if you prefer, lower your gaze to a spot on the floor.
2. **Take a Few Deep Breaths:** Inhale slowly through your nose, filling your belly with air. Exhale slowly through your mouth, releasing any tension.
3. **Focus on Your Breath:** Bring your attention to the sensation of your breath as it enters and leaves your

nostrils or the rise and fall of your chest. Don't try to control your breath; simply observe it.
4. **Notice Your Body:** Scan your body from head to toe, noticing any sensations you feel. Is there tension anywhere? Any areas of relaxation? Simply observe without judgment.
5. **Thoughts Will Come and Go:** It's perfectly normal for thoughts to arise during meditation. Don't judge yourself for having thoughts; simply acknowledge them and gently bring your attention back to your breath or body.
6. **Be Kind to Yourself:** If you find yourself getting distracted or frustrated, don't beat yourself up. Gently redirect your attention back to the present moment. Remember, mindfulness is about being kind to yourself, not critical.
7. **Ending the Meditation:** When your timer goes off, slowly open your eyes or lift your gaze. Take a moment to stretch and notice how you feel.

TIPS FOR A SUCCESSFUL MEDITATION PRACTICE:

- **Consistency is Key:** Aim to meditate daily, even if it's just for a few minutes. Over time, you'll notice a cumulative effect on your well-being.
- **Don't Judge Your Experience:** There's no right or wrong way to meditate. Some days will be easier than others. Simply observe your experience without judgment.

- **Start Small:** If 5 minutes feels too long, start with 2-3 minutes and gradually increase the duration as you get more comfortable.
- **Experiment:** Try different types of meditation, such as guided meditations, walking meditations, or loving-kindness meditations. Find what resonates with you.
- **Create a Sacred Space:** If you have the space, create a dedicated meditation corner with a comfortable cushion, candles, or inspiring objects.
- **Seek Guidance:** If you're struggling with meditation, consider taking a class, attending a retreat, or seeking guidance from a meditation teacher.

THE BENEFITS OF MINDFULNESS:

Practicing mindfulness meditation regularly can have a profound impact on your life. Research has shown that it can:

- **Reduce stress and anxiety:** Mindfulness helps us become more aware of our thoughts and feelings, allowing us to respond to stressors with greater calm and clarity.
- **Improve focus and concentration:** Regular meditation can enhance our ability to concentrate and stay present with tasks.
- **Increase self-awareness:** Mindfulness allows us to observe our thoughts and emotions without judgment, leading to greater self-understanding and acceptance.
- **Cultivate compassion:** By practicing mindfulness, we develop greater compassion for ourselves and others.

- **Enhance overall well-being:** Mindfulness has been linked to improved mood, better sleep, and greater overall happiness.

Remember, mindfulness is not a quick fix; it's a lifelong journey. But with consistent practice, you'll discover its transformative power and experience the many benefits it has to offer. So, take a deep breath, let go of any expectations, and simply be present in this moment.

Day 10: Goal Setting

Welcome to Day 10, where we shift gears from introspection to action. We've spent the past nine days digging deep, confronting fears, and uncovering your purpose. Now, it's time to translate that newfound clarity into concrete goals that will propel you forward.

Think of your goals as a roadmap to your ideal destination – the life you envision for yourself when you've conquered your "what ifs" and embraced your purpose. Without a map, it's easy to wander aimlessly, lose motivation, or get sidetracked by distractions. But with a well-defined plan, you'll have a clear path to follow, milestones to celebrate, and the confidence to keep moving forward, even when the going gets tough.

WHY SETTING GOALS MATTERS

Goals provide direction. They give you a sense of focus and purpose, helping you prioritize your time and energy. Without goals, it's easy to drift through life, reacting to circumstances rather than proactively creating the future you desire.

Goals boost motivation. When you have a clear target in

sight, you're more likely to stay motivated and committed to your journey. The excitement of chasing your dreams and witnessing your progress can be incredibly empowering.

Goals increase self-efficacy. Achieving your goals, big or small, reinforces your belief in your abilities. It proves that you are capable of turning your dreams into reality, which in turn fuels your confidence and resilience.

THE SMART APPROACH TO GOAL SETTING

Not all goals are created equal. Vague, unrealistic, or poorly defined goals can set you up for disappointment and frustration. That's why we'll use the SMART approach to goal setting:

- **Specific:** Your goals should be clear and well-defined. Avoid vague statements like "I want to be happier" and instead focus on specific outcomes like "I want to exercise three times a week" or "I want to start a blog about my passion for photography."
- **Measurable:** Your goals should be quantifiable so you can track your progress and know when you've achieved them. For example, instead of saying "I want to save more money," you could say "I want to save $5,000 for a down payment on a house by the end of the year."
- **Achievable:** Your goals should be challenging yet realistic. Setting unattainable goals can lead to discouragement and demotivation. Start with smaller, more manageable goals and gradually work your way up to bigger ones.

- **Relevant:** Your goals should align with your values, passions, and overall purpose. Don't set goals just because you think you should; choose goals that truly matter to you and will move you closer to the life you desire.
- **Time-Bound:** Your goals should have a deadline or timeframe. This creates a sense of urgency and helps you avoid procrastination. Set realistic deadlines that are challenging but achievable.

FROM PURPOSE TO ACTION

In this chapter, we'll guide you through the process of setting SMART goals that are aligned with your purpose. We'll explore different areas of your life (career, relationships, personal growth, etc.) and help you identify specific goals that will move you closer to your ideal future.

Remember, goal setting isn't just about achieving external success; it's about personal growth, self-discovery, and living a life that is aligned with your deepest values and aspirations. So, let's roll up our sleeves and start mapping out your path to "No More What Ifs!"

SETTING SMART GOALS

Think of your purpose as a destination you're eager to reach. It's
a place where you feel fulfilled, where your passions and talents align with your actions, where you're making a positive impact on the world. But how do you get there? You need

a map, a clear path to follow. That's where SMART goals come in.

SMART goals are like a GPS for your life. They provide the direction and guidance you need to navigate from where you are now to where you want to be. They help you break down your big dreams into manageable steps, ensuring you make progress every day, no matter how small.

WHAT ARE S.M.A.R.T. GOALS?

Let's break down the acronym:

- **Specific:** Your goals should be crystal clear, not vague or general. Instead of saying, "I want to be healthier," say, "I want to run a 5K in three months."
- **Measurable:** You need to be able to track your progress. Instead of saying, "I want to write more," say, "I want to write 500 words every day."
- **Achievable:** Your goals should be challenging but realistic. Don't set yourself up for failure by aiming for something impossible. Instead, set goals that stretch you but are within reach.
- **Relevant:** Your goals should align with your values, passions, and overall purpose. Don't waste time on goals that don't matter to you. Instead, focus on what truly lights you up and moves you closer to your dreams.
- **Time-Bound:** Give yourself a deadline. This creates a sense of urgency and helps you stay motivated. Instead of saying, "I want to learn Spanish," say, "I want to be conversational in Spanish by the end of the year."

WHY ARE SMART GOALS IMPORTANT?

SMART goals are more than just a fancy acronym. They offer a powerful framework for achieving your dreams. Here's why they're so important:

1. **Clarity and Focus:** Vague goals lead to vague results. SMART goals force you to get specific about what you want and how you'll get there. This clarity focuses your energy and eliminates distractions.
2. **Motivation and Accountability:** When your goals are measurable and time-bound, you can easily track your progress. This helps you stay motivated and see how far you've come, even when you face setbacks. It also holds you accountable, making it harder to procrastinate or give up.
3. **Increased Confidence:** As you achieve your SMART goals, your confidence grows. You start to believe in your ability to achieve anything you set your mind to. This increased self-efficacy propels you towards even bigger and bolder goals.
4. **Better Decision Making:** SMART goals provide a framework for making decisions that align with your overall vision. When faced with a choice, you can ask yourself, "Does this move me closer to my goal?" If not, you know it's not the right choice for you.
5. **Reduced Overwhelm:** Big goals can feel overwhelming, but SMART goals break them down into smaller, more manageable steps. This makes them feel less intimidating and more attainable, reducing stress and anxiety.

SETTING SMART GOALS IN ACTION

Remember, setting goals isn't just about writing them down. It's about creating a plan of action and taking consistent steps towards achieving them. Here are a few tips:

- **Write down your goals:** Put them somewhere you'll see them every day. This could be on your vision board, in a journal, or as a phone reminder.
- **Break down big goals:** Divide your goals into smaller, more achievable milestones. This makes them feel less overwhelming and allows you to celebrate your progress along the way.
- **Track your progress:** Use a journal, app, or calendar to track your progress. This will help you stay motivated and make adjustments if needed.
- **Be flexible:** Life happens. Don't beat yourself up if you get off track. Simply adjust your plan and keep moving forward.
- **Celebrate your wins:** Acknowledge and celebrate every victory, no matter how small. This positive reinforcement will keep you motivated and excited about the journey ahead.

Remember, your purpose is a journey, not a destination. Embrace the process of setting and achieving goals, and enjoy the growth and fulfillment that come with living intentionally.

ALIGNING GOALS WITH PURPOSE

Alright, friend, we've unearthed those deep-seated values and passions within you. Now, let's put them to work! It's time to bridge the gap between your aspirations and your actions by setting goals that are in sync with your purpose. Think of it as crafting your personal roadmap to fulfillment.

Picture this: You've got your destination in mind – that's your purpose, your big "why." But how do you get there? You need a map, a route that takes you through exciting landscapes and avoids those dead ends of regret. That's where goal-setting comes in.

PURPOSEFUL GOALS: MORE THAN JUST CHECKMARKS

We've all set goals before. Maybe it was losing those pesky ten pounds, landing a promotion, or finally taking that dream vacation. But how often do we set goals that truly light us up, that make us jump out of bed in the morning, eager to tackle the day?

Purposeful goals are different. They're not just about checking items off a to-do list. They're infused with meaning, driven by your passions, and aligned with your core values. They're the kind of goals that ignite your soul and leave you feeling energized, fulfilled, and deeply satisfied.

Think about it: When your goals are in harmony with your purpose, every step you take feels like a step in the right direction. You're not just working towards an arbitrary achievement; you're living your life in a way that feels authentic and meaningful. You're building a life that you'll look back on with pride and say, "I made a difference. I lived a life that mattered."

THE TRANSFORMATIVE POWER OF PURPOSEFUL GOALS

Purposeful goals have a remarkable way of transforming our lives. They provide us with clarity, focus, and a sense of direction. They motivate us to push past our limits, overcome obstacles, and achieve things we never thought possible.

When our goals are aligned with our purpose, we tap into a deep well of motivation that sustains us through the inevitable challenges and setbacks. We become more resilient, more determined, and more committed to our path. We're no longer driven by external validation or fleeting desires; we're driven by a deep-seated belief in our own potential and the power of our purpose.

Purposeful goals also have a ripple effect on our overall well-being. They boost our self-confidence, increase our happiness levels, and even improve our physical health. When we're living

in alignment with our purpose, we feel a sense of inner peace, joy, and satisfaction that can't be found in external achievements alone.

CRAFTING YOUR PURPOSE-DRIVEN GOALS

Now that you understand the importance of aligning your

goals with your purpose, let's dive into the practical steps for crafting your own purpose-driven goals.

1. **Revisit Your Purpose Statement:** Take a moment to reflect on your purpose statement (you crafted one in Chapter 14, remember?). This statement serves as your North Star, guiding you towards goals that truly matter.
2. **Identify Key Areas of Focus:** Consider the different areas of your life where you want to create change or growth (e.g., career, relationships, personal development, health). Choose 1-3 areas to focus on initially.
3. **Brainstorm Goals That Align with Your Purpose:** Generate a list of potential goals for each area of focus. Ask yourself, "How can I use my passions and talents to achieve these goals? How will these goals contribute to my overall purpose?"
4. **Set SMART Goals:** Make sure your goals are Specific, Measurable, Achievable, Relevant, and Time-Bound. This will help you create a clear roadmap and track your progress.
5. **Break Down Big Goals:** If your goals seem overwhelming, break them down into smaller, more manageable steps. This will make them feel less daunting and more achievable.
6. **Visualize Success:** Create a vivid mental picture of yourself achieving each goal. How will it feel? What will you see, hear, and experience? Visualization can be a powerful motivator.

EMBRACING THE JOURNEY

Remember, setting purposeful goals is not just about the end result. It's about the journey itself. It's about embracing challenges as opportunities for growth, learning from your mistakes, and celebrating your progress along the way.

EXERCISE: GOAL SETTING

Alright, friend, it's time to take all the insights, reflections, and newfound courage you've gathered so far and put them into action. Think of this exercise as crafting a roadmap for your journey ahead – a roadmap guided by your purpose and designed to lead you to a life of "no more what ifs."

Remember those SMART goals we talked about? Specific, Measurable, Achievable, Relevant, and Time-Bound? They're not just a fancy acronym; they're a powerful framework for turning your dreams into reality. Let's put them to work.

Step 1: Reflect and Refine

Take a moment to revisit the "What If" Inventory and the Fear and Regret Journal you completed earlier. What fears or regrets are holding you back the most? What aspirations are calling to you the loudest? Choose 1-3 areas where you want to see significant growth or change.

Step 2: Get SMART

For each area you've chosen, let's craft a SMART goal:

- **Specific:** What exactly do you want to achieve? Be as clear and detailed as possible. Instead of "I want to be healthier," try "I want to lose 10 pounds and run a 5k in six months."
- **Measurable:** How will you know you've achieved your goal? What specific metrics or milestones can you track? For example, instead of "I want to improve my relationships," try "I want to have one meaningful conversation with a friend each week."
- **Achievable:** Is your goal realistic and attainable given your current resources and circumstances? If your goal feels overwhelming, break it down into smaller, more manageable steps.
- **Relevant:** Does your goal align with your values, passions, and purpose? Will achieving it bring you closer to the life you envision?
- **Time-Bound:** When do you want to achieve this goal? Setting a deadline creates a sense of urgency and helps you stay focused.

Step 3: Break It Down

Once you have your SMART goals, it's time to break them down into smaller, actionable steps. This is where the rubber meets the road. Instead of focusing on the overwhelming end goal, concentrate on the daily or weekly actions that will move you closer to it.

Let's say your goal is to write a book. Instead of thinking, "I need to write a whole book," break it down into manageable tasks like:

- Write 500 words a day.
- Research for 30 minutes a day.
- Outline one chapter per week.

These smaller steps make the goal seem less daunting and more achievable. You can track your progress, celebrate your milestones, and adjust your approach as needed.

Example: Overcoming the Fear of Public Speaking

Let's say you've identified a fear of public speaking as a major obstacle in your life. Here's how you could create a SMART goal and break it down into actionable steps:

- **Specific:** I want to be able to deliver a 10-minute presentation to a group of 20 people without feeling overwhelmed by anxiety.
- **Measurable:** I will practice my presentation in front of a mirror or with a friend twice a week.
- **Achievable:** I will start by practicing in front of one or two people and gradually increase the audience size.
- **Relevant:** This goal is relevant because it aligns with my desire to share my expertise and make a difference in the world.
- **Time-Bound:** I will achieve this goal within three months.

Actionable Steps:

- Week 1-2: Practice the presentation in front of a mirror or with a supportive friend.
- Week 3-4: Deliver the presentation to a small group of 3-5 people.
- Week 5-6: Deliver the presentation to a larger group of 10 people.
- Week 7-8: Continue practicing and refining the presentation.
- Week 9-12: Deliver the presentation to a group of 20 people.

By breaking down this seemingly daunting goal into smaller, manageable steps, you make it feel less overwhelming and more attainable. You can track your progress, celebrate your successes, and build your confidence along the way.

Remember:

- **Be Flexible:** Your goals may evolve as you progress, and that's okay. Allow yourself the flexibility to adjust your plan as needed.
- **Celebrate Progress:** Don't just focus on the end goal. Celebrate every small win along the way to keep yourself motivated and on track.
- **Don't Give Up:** There will be setbacks and challenges, but don't let them derail you. Persevere, learn from your mistakes, and keep moving forward.

By setting SMART goals and breaking them down into actionable steps, you're not just dreaming about a better future; you're actively creating it. This is your roadmap to a life of "no more what ifs." So, grab your pen, start planning, and get ready to embrace a life filled with purpose, passion, and possibility.

Part 2: Embracing Your Purpose (Days 11-20)

Day 11: Discovering Your "Why"

Up to this point, we've tackled the shadows of fear and regret, and you've started building a toolkit for a more positive and empowered mindset. Now, it's time to delve into the heart of what truly drives you: your "why."

You may have heard the saying, "Do what you love, and you'll never work a day in your life." While there's truth to the idea of finding joy in our work, it's important to understand that purpose goes beyond simply doing what we enjoy. It's about connecting our passions to a deeper sense of meaning and contribution.

Think of it this way: passion is the fuel, but purpose is the engine. Passion provides the initial spark and excitement, but purpose gives us the direction, the endurance, and the resilience to keep going, even when faced with challenges.

Discovering your "why" is like finding your North Star. It's a guiding principle that helps you navigate life's twists and turns, make decisions that align with your values, and create a meaningful impact on the world.

VALUES: YOUR INNER COMPASS

Your values are the fundamental beliefs that guide your actions and choices. They are the things that matter most to you, the principles you hold dear. When you live in alignment with your values, you feel a sense of integrity, authenticity, and fulfillment.

Discovering your "why" often involves identifying your core values. These values are the foundation upon which your purpose is built. They provide the framework for understanding what truly motivates you, what you stand for, and how you want to contribute to the world.

Think about it:

- *What are the qualities you admire most in others?*
- *What causes are you passionate about supporting?*
- *What brings you the most joy and fulfillment in life?*
- *What kind of legacy do you want to leave behind?*

By answering these questions and exploring your values, you'll gain clarity and direction in discovering your "why." You'll begin to see how your passions and talents can be used to serve a greater purpose, one that aligns with your deepest beliefs and values.

This chapter will guide you through a values assessment exercise to help you identify your core values. Once you know what truly matters to you, you'll be equipped to make choices that are in alignment with your purpose and create a life that feels meaningful and fulfilling.

So let's dive in and explore the values that light your path. Your "why" is waiting to be discovered.

BEYOND PASSION

Let's be honest: the idea of finding your passion and turning it into your life's work sounds amazing. Who wouldn't want to spend their days doing what they love? But let's dig a little deeper. Passion is a wonderful starting point, but it's not the entire picture. Purpose goes beyond simply doing what you enjoy. It's about connecting those passions to a deeper sense of meaning and contribution. It's about finding your "why."

Think of it this way: passion is the fuel, but purpose is the steering wheel. Passion gives you the energy and enthusiasm to get going, but purpose gives you direction. It's the compass that guides you through life's twists and turns, helping you make decisions that align with your values and aspirations.

PASSION VS. PURPOSE: A KEY DISTINCTION

Passion is often associated with excitement, enjoyment, and a sense of flow. When you're passionate about something, time seems to fly by, and you feel fully engaged in the moment. It's that feeling of "I could do this all day!"

Purpose, on the other hand, is about impact. It's the answer to the question "Why does this matter?" It's the reason you get out of bed in the morning, the driving force behind your actions, and the legacy you want to leave behind.

While passion can certainly be a part of your purpose,

it's not the sole defining factor. You can be passionate about baking delicious cakes, but your purpose might be to use your baking skills to bring joy to others, create a community gathering space, or support a local charity.

IDENTIFYING YOUR "WHY"

So, how do you discover your "why"? It's a personal journey of self-reflection and exploration. Here are some questions to ponder:

- **What are your core values?** What principles are most important to you? What kind of impact do you want to have on the world?
- **What are your unique strengths and talents?** What are you naturally good at? What skills and abilities do you possess that could benefit others?
- **What problems or challenges do you care deeply about?** Are there any causes or issues that you feel passionate about addressing?
- **What makes you feel most alive and fulfilled?** What activities or experiences bring you the most joy and satisfaction?

Take some time to reflect on these questions. Journal about them, meditate on them, or discuss them with a trusted friend or mentor. The answers may not come immediately, but as you delve deeper into your inner world, you'll start to see patterns emerge. You'll begin to connect the dots between your passions, values, and strengths, and a clearer sense of purpose will begin to take shape.

THE POWER OF PURPOSE

Once you've identified your "why," it becomes a powerful source of motivation and resilience. It fuels your drive, keeps you focused on your goals, and helps you overcome obstacles.

Think of a time when you faced a major challenge in your life. What kept you going? Was it a deep-seated belief in the importance of what you were doing? A desire to make a difference? A sense of responsibility to yourself or others? That's your purpose at work.

When you're connected to your "why," setbacks become learning opportunities, not failures. Challenges become fuel for growth, not reasons to quit. You develop a resilience that allows you to bounce back from adversity and continue moving forward.

In the next section, we'll explore how your passion and purpose intersect to create a fulfilling and meaningful life. We'll discuss how to align your actions with your "why" and how to use your unique gifts to make a positive impact on the world. So stay tuned, because your journey to purpose is just beginning!

THE POWER OF VALUES

Let's talk about values. You've probably heard this word thrown around, but what does it really mean? And why are values so important when it comes to living a purposeful, regret-free life?

Think of your values as your inner compass. They are the deeply held beliefs that guide your actions, decisions, and how you show up in the world. They act as a filter, helping you discern what's truly important to you and what's not.

When your actions align with your values, you feel a sense of integrity and authenticity. You're not just going through the motions; you're living in a way that feels true to who you are. This alignment brings a sense of peace, fulfillment, and joy.

But when your actions clash with your values, it creates internal conflict and dissonance. You may feel stressed, unhappy, or even resentful. You might start to question your choices and wonder if you're on the right path.

That's why it's crucial to identify and clarify your core values. They are the foundation upon which you build a life of purpose, meaning, and fulfillment.

WHAT ARE YOUR CORE VALUES?

Core values are the non-negotiables in your life. They are the principles that you hold most dear, the ones that shape your character and guide your behavior. They are the qualities that you strive to embody, the things that make you feel alive and authentic.

Your core values might include:

- **Integrity:** Being honest, ethical, and true to your word

- **Compassion:** Showing empathy and kindness towards others
- **Growth:** Continuously learning, evolving, and challenging yourself
- **Authenticity:** Being genuine and true to yourself
- **Courage:** Facing your fears and taking risks
- **Creativity:** Expressing yourself through art, music, writing, or other creative outlets
- **Connection:** Building meaningful relationships with others
- **Service:** Contributing to your community or the world at large
- **Adventure:** Seeking out new experiences and embracing the unknown

This is just a small sample of possible values. Your core values will be unique to you, based on your personal experiences, beliefs, and aspirations.

HOW TO IDENTIFY YOUR CORE VALUES

There are many ways to uncover your core values. Here are a few exercises you can try:

1. **Reflect on Peak Experiences:** Think back to times in your life when you felt most alive, joyful, and fulfilled. What values were present in those moments?
2. **Consider Your Role Models:** Who do you admire most, and what qualities do they embody? What values do you resonate with in them?

3. **Examine Your Reactions:** Pay attention to how you react to different situations. What makes you feel angry, frustrated, or inspired? These emotional responses can be clues to your underlying values.
4. **Create a Values List:** Write down a list of words that resonate with you (e.g., honesty, courage, kindness, creativity). Then, narrow down the list to your top 5-10 most important values.
5. **Prioritize Your Values:** Rank your values in order of importance. This will help you clarify what truly matters most to you.

Once you've identified your core values, it's important to integrate them into your daily life. Use them as a filter for decision-making. When faced with a choice, ask yourself, "Does this align with my values?" If the answer is no, reconsider your options.

Your values can also guide your goals and aspirations. What kind of life do you want to create? What impact do you want to have on the world? When your goals are rooted in your values, they become more meaningful and fulfilling.

Remember, your values may evolve and change over time. As you grow and learn, you may discover new values or re-prioritize existing ones. That's okay! The key is to be intentional about checking in with your values regularly and making sure your choices are aligned with what truly matters to you.

By understanding and living by your core values, you create a solid foundation for a life of purpose, passion, and regret-free living. You'll make decisions with confidence, knowing that you're staying true to your authentic self. And that's the most powerful way to create a life you love.

EXERCISE: VALUES ASSESSMENT

Alright, friend, it's time to roll up our sleeves and get to the heart of what truly matters to you. Remember, living with intention means aligning your actions with your values. But first, we need to uncover those values—those guiding principles that light up your soul and give your life meaning.

Think of your values as your inner compass. They point you in the right direction, helping you make choices that feel authentic and fulfilling. When you're living in alignment with your values, life feels more harmonious, and you're less likely to experience regrets.

Let's dive into a values assessment exercise to uncover your core values. Don't worry; there are no right or wrong answers here. This is about YOU, your unique essence, and what makes your heart sing.

Step 1: Gather Your Tools Grab a pen, a notebook, and a comfortable spot where you can reflect without distractions. You can also download a printable values list from our website (insert link) or simply use the following list as a starting point:

- Authenticity
- Adventure
- Balance
- Compassion
- Creativity

- Courage
- Family
- Financial Security
- Freedom
- Friendship
- Fun
- Growth
- Health
- Honesty
- Integrity
- Joy
- Kindness
- Leadership
- Learning
- Love
- Loyalty
- Openness
- Optimism
- Peace
- Personal Development
- Respect
- Spirituality
- Stability
- Success
- Trustworthiness

Feel free to add any other values that resonate with you.

Step 2: Identify Your Top Values Look over the list of values and circle any that jump out at you. Don't overthink it.

Go with your gut reaction. Aim to circle around 15-20 values that feel most meaningful to you.

Now, here comes the slightly tricky part. From your circled values, choose your top 10. This may require some careful consideration. Think about which values are most important to you, the ones that guide your decisions and actions most often.

Step 3: Rank Your Top Values Take your top 10 values and rank them in order of importance, from most important (#1) to least important (#10). This can be a bit challenging, as all of your values are likely meaningful to you. But trust your intuition and see what emerges.

Step 4: Reflect on Your Values Take a deep breath and review your top 10 values. These are the guiding principles that shape your life. They are the qualities you strive for, the things that bring you joy and fulfillment.

Now, ask yourself the following questions:

- *How do these values show up in my life currently? Are there specific examples of times when I've lived in alignment with these values?*
- *Are there any values that I'm not fully living by? Why might that be? Are there any obstacles or fears holding me back?*
- *What would it look like to live more fully in alignment with these values? What changes could I make in my daily life, my relationships, or my career?*
- *How can I use my values as a compass to guide me towards my purpose and a life of "no more what ifs"?*

Take your time to reflect on these questions. Write down your thoughts, feelings, and any insights that arise. This is a powerful exercise for self-discovery and creating a life that is authentically yours.

Remember, your values aren't set in stone. They can evolve and change as you grow and evolve. The important thing is to be aware of them and to use them as a tool for making intentional choices that lead you towards a fulfilling life.

This values assessment exercise is just the beginning of your journey towards living with intention. Keep these values close to your heart as we move forward, as they will serve as a guiding light throughout this book and beyond.

Day 12: Passion Meets Purpose

Think back to a time when you felt truly alive, energized, and completely absorbed in what you were doing. Maybe it was losing yourself in a creative project, volunteering for a cause you care about, or simply sharing a laugh with a loved one. Whatever it was, chances are it tapped into something deeper within you – your passions.

Today, we're going to explore the powerful connection between passion and purpose. We'll delve into how your passions can be harnessed to not only bring you joy but also to serve others and make a positive impact on the world.

MORE THAN JUST A HOBBY

Passion isn't just about hobbies or passing interests. It's that spark of excitement, that feeling of flow that makes time melt away. It's that thing that makes you say, "I love doing this!"

But passion is also a powerful force that can fuel our purpose. When we align our actions with our passions, we tap into a wellspring of energy, motivation, and resilience. We become more engaged, more focused, and more determined to overcome obstacles.

THE INTERSECTION OF PASSION AND SERVICE

Think of your passions as clues to your purpose. They reveal what truly matters to you, what lights you up, and what you're naturally drawn to. When you use your passions in service of others, you create a powerful synergy that not only benefits the world but also brings you a deep sense of fulfillment.

Consider the musician who uses their talent to bring joy to audiences, the teacher who inspires a love of learning in their students, or the entrepreneur who creates a product that solves a real problem. These are just a few examples of how passion and purpose can intersect to create meaningful impact.

YOUR UNIQUE CONTRIBUTION

You have unique gifts and talents that the world needs. Your passions are not just for you; they're meant to be shared. When you use your passions to contribute to something bigger than yourself, you tap into a deeper sense of meaning and purpose.

Maybe you're a natural storyteller who can use your words to inspire and uplift others. Maybe you're a skilled problem-solver who can create innovative solutions to challenges.

Maybe you're a compassionate listener who can offer support and guidance to those in need. Whatever your passions may be, there are countless ways to use them to make a difference.

TODAY'S CHALLENGE: TAKE PURPOSEFUL ACTION

Today, I challenge you to take one small step towards aligning your passion with your purpose. It doesn't have to be anything grand or life-changing. It could be as simple as volunteering

your time for a cause you care about, starting a blog to share your knowledge, or simply offering a helping hand to someone in need.

Remember, every small step you take towards living your purpose is a victory. It's a way to honor your passions, contribute to the world, and create a life that is both fulfilling and meaningful.

THE INTERSECTION OF PASSION AND SERVICE

Think back to Day 8 when we explored your passions – those activities, hobbies, or causes that light you up from the inside out. Now, let's dive deeper into how those passions can be harnessed for a greater purpose. Because here's the secret: your passions aren't just meant for your own enjoyment; they're powerful tools for serving others and making a positive impact on the world.

I know it may sound a bit idealistic but hear me out. Your

passions hold a unique potential. They're not just random interests; they're clues to your innate talents, your unique gifts, and your potential to contribute to something bigger than yourself.

When you combine your passion with a desire to serve others, something magical happens. Your work becomes more than just a job; it becomes a calling. Your efforts feel less like a chore and more like a contribution. You tap into a deeper sense of meaning and fulfillment, knowing that what you're doing matters.

THE PASSION-PURPOSE CONNECTION

Let's face it: we all want to feel like our lives have significance. We yearn to make a difference, leave a mark, and create something that outlasts us. But sometimes, we get caught up in the daily grind, chasing external validation, or simply trying to survive. We forget to connect with what truly matters to us.

That's where passion comes in. It's a compass pointing us towards our true north. When we follow our passions, we're not just doing things we enjoy; we're tapping into our inherent strengths and talents. We're unlocking our potential to create, contribute, and connect with others in a meaningful way.

Think of your passion as a gift you've been given. It's something you're naturally good at, something that excites and energizes you. But like any gift, it's not meant to be hoarded; it's meant to be shared. When you share your passion with the world, you're not just giving of yourself; you're also receiving the joy, satisfaction, and fulfillment that comes from making a positive impact.

FROM PASSION TO PURPOSEFUL ACTION

You might be wondering, "How do I turn my passion into something that serves others?" The answer lies in finding the intersection between what you love and what the world needs.

Think about the problems you see in your community or the world at large. What causes do you care about? What skills and talents do you have that could be used to address these issues? How can your passion help make a difference?

Let me share a few examples to spark your imagination:

- **The Artist with a Cause:** Imagine an artist who is passionate about environmental conservation. They use their artistic talents to create paintings that raise awareness about climate change, donate a portion of their profits to environmental organizations, or even lead art workshops that encourage others to connect with nature.
- **The Entrepreneur with a Social Mission:** Picture an entrepreneur who loves technology but is also deeply concerned about educational inequality. They create a startup that develops affordable educational software for underserved communities, providing access to quality learning resources for those who need it most.
- **The Teacher Who Inspires Change:** Consider a teacher who is passionate about social justice. They create a curriculum that teaches students about diversity, inclusion, and equity. They also empower their students to take action in their communities, inspiring the next generation of changemakers.

These are just a few examples, but the possibilities are endless. No matter what your passion is, there's likely a way to connect it to a greater purpose. You might volunteer your time to a cause you care about, use your skills to help others, or even create a business that makes a positive impact.

Remember, you don't have to quit your job or start a non-profit to live a purposeful life. It's about finding ways to integrate your passions into your daily life and making choices that align with your values. It's about using your unique gifts to contribute to something bigger than yourself.

So, take some time to reflect on your passions and how they might be used to serve others. What problems do you see in the world that you want to solve? What skills and talents do you have that could be of use? How can you turn your passion into a force for good? The answers to these questions will lead you closer to your purpose and a life of "no more what ifs."

FINDING YOUR UNIQUE CONTRIBUTION

Now that you've explored your passions, values, and strengths, it's time to delve deeper into how you can make a unique contribution to the world.

Think of it like this: your passions are your fuel, your values are your compass, and your strengths are your tools. Now, you need to find the right "building site" where you can use these resources to create something meaningful.

Your unique contribution lies at the intersection of your passions and the needs of the world. It's about finding a way to use your talents and skills to make a positive impact, whether it's big or small.

LOOK FOR PROBLEMS TO SOLVE

One of the most powerful ways to find your unique contribution is to look for problems that need solving. What issues or challenges resonate with you? What are you naturally curious about? What breaks your heart or gets you fired up?

It could be a local issue, like food insecurity in your community, or a global problem, like climate change. It could be a social issue, like inequality or discrimination, or a personal struggle, like overcoming addiction or mental illness.

Your passion for a particular issue is often a sign that you have a unique perspective or skillset to offer. Maybe you have a knack for organizing, so you could start a local food drive or volunteer at a homeless shelter. Maybe you're a talented writer, so you could raise awareness about social justice issues through your words. Or perhaps you have a gift for listening, so you could offer support to those struggling with addiction.

EXPLORE YOUR INTERESTS

Another way to discover your unique contribution is to explore your interests and hobbies. What activities make you lose track of time? What do you love to learn about? What are you naturally good at?

Your interests often hold clues about your hidden talents and potential contributions. For example, if you love to cook, maybe you could teach cooking classes to underprivileged youth or start a catering business that supports sustainable agriculture. If you're passionate about animals, maybe you could volunteer at an animal shelter, become a pet therapist, or advocate for animal rights.

Remember, your contribution doesn't have to be grandiose or world-changing. Even small acts of kindness and service can make a significant impact on the lives of others.

Ask Yourself Key Questions

To help you identify your unique contribution, ask yourself these key questions:

- *What am I naturally good at?*
- *What do I enjoy doing?*
- *What problems or needs do I see in the world?*
- *How can I use my skills and passions to address those needs?*
- *What unique perspective or experience can I offer?*
- *What kind of impact do I want to make?*

Don't be afraid to experiment and try different things. Your unique contribution may not be immediately obvious, but through exploration and self-reflection, you'll eventually find your niche.

CONNECT WITH YOUR COMMUNITY

Talk to friends, family, and mentors about your interests and passions. They may have insights or connections that can help you find opportunities to contribute. Look for volunteer opportunities, internships, or jobs that align with your values and goals.

Remember, your unique contribution is not something

you find; it's something you create. It's the result of your passions, your values, your skills, and your willingness to make a difference. So get out there, explore, experiment, and discover how you can use your unique gifts to make the world a better place.

EXERCISE: THE "I CAN" LIST

1. Take a sheet of paper and write down all the things you can do. This could include skills, talents, hobbies, or any other abilities you possess.
2. Next, think about the problems or needs you see in your community or the world.
3. Look for overlaps between your "I Can" list and the needs you identified. Are there any ways you could use your skills or passions to address those needs?
4. Brainstorm specific actions you could take to make a contribution, no matter how small.

This exercise will help you identify your unique strengths and how you can use them to create positive change in the world. Remember, your contribution doesn't have to be perfect or groundbreaking. It simply needs to come from your heart and be aligned with your passions and values.

EXERCISE: PURPOSEFUL ACTS

You've spent the past few days delving into your passions, values, and purpose. You've crafted a vision for your future and started to envision the impact you want to make on the world. Now, it's time to translate that vision into action.

Remember, living a purposeful life isn't just about grand gestures or major milestones. It's about infusing intention and meaning into your everyday choices. It's about taking small, consistent steps that align with your values and move you closer to your goals.

That's where purposeful acts come in. These are intentional actions, big or small, that reflect your passions and values. They're not about adding more to your to-do list; they're about making choices that feel authentic and meaningful to you.

Purposeful acts can take many forms:

- **Volunteering your time:** Is there a cause you care about? A local organization that could use your help? Volunteering is a powerful way to give back to your community and make a difference in the lives of others.
- **Starting a passion project:** Have you always wanted to write a book, learn a new language, or start a blog? Don't let fear or procrastination hold you back. Take that first step and begin exploring your passions.
- **Helping someone in need:** Look for opportunities to lend a helping hand to those around you. It could be as simple as offering a listening ear, running an errand for a neighbor, or donating to a charity you support.
- **Expressing your creativity:** Do you love to paint, write, sing, or dance? Find ways to express your creativity and share your talents with the world.
- **Connecting with loved ones:** Spend quality time

with family and friends. Deepen your relationships and create meaningful connections.
- **Taking care of yourself:** Prioritize your physical and mental well-being. Engage in activities that nourish your soul and recharge your batteries.

BRAINSTORMING YOUR PURPOSEFUL ACT

Now, it's your turn to brainstorm and plan your own purposeful act. Take out your journal or a piece of paper and start exploring these questions:

1. **What am I passionate about?** What topics, activities, or causes ignite your enthusiasm and energy?
2. **What are my core values?** What principles are most important to you in life? How can you express these values through your actions?
3. **What impact do I want to make?** How can you use your passions and values to contribute to the world around you?

Don't overthink it. Let your intuition guide you. Write down any ideas that come to mind, no matter how big or small.

Planning Your Action

Once you've brainstormed a few ideas, choose one purposeful act that resonates with you the most. Then, create a plan for how you will take action.

Your plan should include:

- **Specific action steps:** Break down your purposeful act into smaller, manageable steps.
- **Timeline:** Set a realistic timeline for completing each step.
- **Resources:** Identify any resources you might need, such as materials, information, or support from others.
- **Obstacles:** Anticipate any potential obstacles or challenges and brainstorm solutions.

Remember, this is your personal journey. There's no right or wrong way to take action. Choose something that feels exciting, meaningful, and aligned with your values.

Taking the First Step

Now that you have a plan in place, it's time to take the first step. Don't let fear or self-doubt hold you back. Remember, even small actions can have a big impact.

As you take action, pay attention to how you feel. Does this purposeful act bring you joy, fulfillment, and a sense of purpose? If so, you're on the right track. If not, don't be afraid to adjust your plan or try something different.

The most important thing is to keep moving forward, one step at a time. By taking consistent action aligned with your passions and values, you'll start to build momentum and create a life that is rich in purpose and meaning.

So go out there and make a difference! The world needs your unique gifts and talents.

Day 13: Clarifying Your Vision

Ever get that feeling of being lost in a fog, unsure of which path to take? Maybe you have a vague sense of what you want, but the details are fuzzy, like a picture slightly out of focus. That's where clarifying your vision comes in.

Think of your vision as a compass, a guiding star that points you towards your true north. It's the mental picture of the life you want to create, the goals you want to achieve, and the impact you want to have on the world. When your vision is clear, it becomes a powerful motivator, propelling you forward and helping you make decisions aligned with your deepest desires.

So, why is clarifying your vision so important on this journey to living a regret-free life?

First, a clear vision gives you direction. It's like having a map that shows you the way, preventing you from wandering aimlessly or getting sidetracked by distractions. When you know where you're headed, it's easier to say "no" to things that don't serve your purpose and "yes" to opportunities that align with your goals.

Second, a clear vision ignites your motivation. When you can vividly picture the life you want to create, it becomes a source of inspiration and excitement. It fuels your passion, keeps you focused, and helps you push through challenges.

Third, a clear vision empowers you to make better choices. When faced with decisions, you can ask yourself, "Does this align with my vision?" If not, you can confidently choose a different path. This helps you avoid decisions you might later regret.

Finally, a clear vision fosters resilience. When setbacks inevitably arise, your vision acts as an anchor, reminding you of the bigger picture and your ultimate goals. It helps you bounce back from challenges with renewed determination and focus.

Today, we're going to delve into the power of visualization and learn how to create a vision board that brings your dreams to life. This isn't about wishful thinking or unrealistic fantasies; it's about harnessing the power of your mind to create a compelling picture of the future you want to manifest.

By the end of today, you'll have a clear vision for your life and a tangible tool to help you stay focused and motivated. So let's get started on this exciting step towards a life of purpose, passion, and no regrets.

THE POWER OF VISUALIZATION

Close your eyes for a moment and imagine your ideal life. Picture yourself achieving your biggest goals, living your dreams, and experiencing the joy and fulfillment you deeply desire. What do you see? What do you feel? This is the power of visualization.

Visualization isn't just wishful thinking; it's a powerful tool backed by science and utilized by successful people across various fields. It involves creating a vivid mental picture of your desired outcomes, engaging all your senses to make it as real as possible.

But why is visualization so effective? How can simply imagining something make it more likely to happen?

THE SCIENCE BEHIND VISUALIZATION

Visualization works by tapping into the incredible power of our minds. Our brains often struggle to distinguish between vividly imagined experiences and real ones. When we visualize ourselves achieving our goals, our brains fire up the same neural pathways as if we were actually experiencing those successes.

This has a profound impact on our motivation, confidence, and decision-making:

- **Increased Motivation:** When we visualize ourselves achieving our goals, we get a taste of the positive emotions associated with success. This surge of excitement and anticipation fuels our motivation, making us more likely to take action towards our dreams.
- **Boosted Confidence:** Visualization helps us build a strong sense of self-efficacy – the belief in our ability to succeed. By repeatedly seeing ourselves overcoming

challenges and achieving our goals, we develop the confidence to take risks and persevere through setbacks.
- **Improved Decision-Making:** Visualization helps us clarify our priorities and make choices that align with our goals. By picturing the different paths we could take, we can assess potential outcomes and make more informed decisions.
- **Reduced Anxiety and Stress:** Visualization can also help us manage stress and anxiety by creating a mental image of a calm and successful outcome. This can be particularly helpful when facing challenging situations or preparing for important events.

VISUALIZATION IN ACTION: REAL-WORLD EXAMPLES

The power of visualization isn't just theoretical; it's been proven time and again by successful individuals across various fields:

- Athletes use visualization to enhance their performance, imagining themselves executing perfect movements and achieving victory.
- Entrepreneurs visualize their businesses thriving, attracting customers, and reaching financial goals.
- Artists visualize their creative process, envisioning the finished product before putting brush to canvas or pen to paper.

Even in everyday life, visualization can be a powerful tool.

Imagine yourself acing a job interview, delivering a confident presentation, or having a difficult conversation with grace and ease. By visualizing success, you set yourself up for a positive outcome.

HOW TO HARNESS THE POWER OF VISUALIZATION

Here are some practical tips for incorporating visualization into your daily routine:

1. **Get Clear on Your Goals:** Before you can visualize your success, you need to know what you're aiming for. Get specific about your goals, whether they're related to your career, relationships, health, or personal growth.
2. **Create a Vivid Mental Picture:** Close your eyes and imagine yourself achieving your goal. Engage all your senses – what do you see, hear, feel, smell, and taste? The more vivid and detailed your visualization, the more impactful it will be.
3. **Practice Regularly:** Visualization is like a muscle – the more you use it, the stronger it gets. Set aside a few minutes each day to visualize your goals, whether it's first thing in the morning, before bed, or during a quiet moment in your day.
4. **Feel the Emotions:** As you visualize, allow yourself to feel the positive emotions associated with success. This will reinforce the neural connections in your brain and make your vision even more powerful.
5. **Take Action:** Visualization is not a substitute for

action, but it can be a powerful catalyst. Use the motivation and confidence you gain from visualizing to take concrete steps toward your goals.

Remember, visualization is a personal practice. There's no right or wrong way to do it. Experiment with different techniques and find what works best for you. The key is to be consistent and to believe in the power of your mind to create the reality you desire.

CREATING A VISION BOARD

Have you ever heard the saying, "A picture is worth a thousand words"? When it comes to our goals and aspirations, this couldn't be more true. That's where the power of a vision board comes in.

What is a Vision Board?

Think of a vision board as a collage of your dreams. It's a visual representation of your goals, desires, and the life you want to create. It can be a physical board filled with magazine clippings, photos, quotes, and drawings, or a digital creation using online tools or apps. The key is to fill it with images and words that evoke the feelings and experiences you want to attract into your life.

Why Create a Vision Board?

A vision board isn't just a fun craft project; it's a powerful tool for manifestation and personal growth. Here's why:

1. **Clarifies Your Vision:** It forces you to get specific about your goals and dreams. Instead of vague aspirations,

you'll be able to visualize exactly what you want to achieve.

2. **Increases Motivation:** Seeing your dreams on display every day serves as a constant reminder of what you're working towards. It can reignite your passion and keep you motivated, especially when faced with challenges.
3. **Enhances Focus:** A vision board helps you prioritize what's truly important to you. By focusing on your vision, you're more likely to make decisions and take actions that align with your goals.
4. **Strengthens Belief:** When you see your dreams in front of you, they start to feel more tangible and achievable. This can boost your confidence and strengthen your belief in your ability to make them a reality.
5. **Attracts Opportunities:** Some believe that a vision board can act as a magnet for opportunities and resources that support your goals. By visualizing what you want, you may start to notice synchronicities and open doors that lead you closer to your dreams.

HOW TO CREATE YOUR VISION BOARD

Creating a vision board is a personal and creative process. There are no right or wrong ways to do it. The most important thing is

to have fun and let your intuition guide you. Here are some steps to get you started:

1. **Gather Your Supplies:** If you're creating a physical vision board, you'll need a board (poster board,

corkboard, etc.), magazines, scissors, glue, markers, and any other decorative materials you like. For a digital vision board, you can use online tools like Canva, Pinterest, or Milanote.

2. **Set Your Intentions:** Before you start, take a few moments to reflect on what you truly want to create in your life. Think about your goals, dreams, and aspirations in different areas of your life (career, relationships, health, personal growth, etc.).
3. **Start Collecting:** Flip through magazines, browse online images, or create your own drawings and artwork. Look for images, words, and quotes that resonate with your vision and evoke positive emotions.
4. **Get Creative:** Start arranging your images and words on your board in a way that feels visually appealing and inspiring to you. There are no rules here – let your creativity flow!
5. **Add Personal Touches:** Make your vision board truly yours by adding personal touches like photos, mementos, or handwritten affirmations.
6. **Display Your Creation:** Place your vision board somewhere you'll see it every day, such as your bedroom, office, or bathroom mirror. This will serve as a daily reminder of your dreams and goals.

TIPS FOR MAKING YOUR VISION BOARD WORK FOR YOU

- **Be Specific:** Instead of using generic images, choose

ones that represent your specific goals (e.g., a photo of your dream house, not just any house).
- **Include Emotions:** Choose images and words that evoke positive emotions (e.g., joy, excitement, gratitude). This will help you connect with your vision on a deeper level.
- **Keep it Updated:** Your vision board is not set in stone. As your goals and dreams evolve, feel free to update and revise your board.
- **Take Action:** A vision board is not a magic wand. It's a tool to help you clarify your vision and stay motivated. Remember to take action steps towards your goals every day.

Your vision board is a powerful tool for turning your dreams into reality. Use it as a daily reminder of what's possible for you, and let it inspire you to take action and create the life you truly desire.

EXERCISE: VISION BOARD CREATION

Ready to turn your dreams into reality? Let's get creative and start building your vision board! This isn't just a fun arts and
crafts project; it's a powerful tool to visualize your goals, reinforce your intentions, and manifest the life you desire.

WHAT'S A VISION BOARD?

Think of your vision board as a collage of your dreams. It's a visual representation of your goals, aspirations, and the life you want to create. It can include images, words, quotes, and anything else that inspires and motivates you.

WHY CREATE A VISION BOARD?

- **Clarity:** A vision board helps you gain clarity on what you truly want in life. By focusing on specific images and words, you define your goals and desires more concretely.
- **Motivation:** Seeing your vision board daily reminds you of what you're working towards, keeping you motivated and inspired.
- **Focus:** Your vision board acts as a visual anchor, helping you focus your energy and attention on what truly matters.
- **Manifestation:** Many people believe that vision boards can help manifest their dreams by aligning their thoughts and actions with their desires.

Gather Your Supplies:

- A large poster board or corkboard
- Magazines, newspapers, or printed images
- Scissors
- Glue or tape
- Markers, colored pencils, or paint (optional)
- Any other decorative items you'd like to use

Step 1: Brainstorm Your Vision Before you start cutting

and pasting, take some time to brainstorm your vision for the future. Think about all areas of your life:

- **Personal Growth:** What skills do you want to develop? What kind of person do you want to become?
- **Career:** What do you want to achieve professionally? What kind of work environment do you desire?
- **Relationships:** What kind of relationships do you want to cultivate? How do you want to feel loved and supported?
- **Health & Wellness:** What are your fitness goals? How do you envision your overall well-being?
- **Finances:** What are your financial aspirations? What kind of lifestyle do you want to create?
- **Fun & Adventure:** What experiences do you want to have? Where do you want to travel?
- **Spirituality:** How do you want to connect with your spirituality or faith?

Step 2: Find Images and Words Now, start browsing through magazines, newspapers, or online image libraries. Look for images, words, and quotes that resonate with your vision. Don't overthink it—let your intuition guide you.

Tips for Finding Images:

- Look for images that evoke strong emotions in you.
- Choose images that represent the feelings you want to experience in your life.
- Don't limit yourself to literal representations. Abstract images can be just as powerful.

Step 3: Start Assembling Your Vision Board Once you have a good collection of images and words, it's time to start assembling your vision board. There are no right or wrong ways to do this. Have fun with it and let your creativity flow!

TIPS FOR ASSEMBLING YOUR VISION BOARD:

- Arrange the images and words in a way that feels visually appealing to you.
- Use different sizes and shapes to create a dynamic layout.
- Add your own personal touches, such as handwritten notes, drawings, or decorations.
- Leave some blank space to allow for new additions or changes over time.

Step 4: Activating Your Vision Board Your vision board is more than just a pretty picture. It's a tool for manifesting your dreams into reality. Here are some ways to activate your vision board:

- Place it somewhere you'll see it every day.
- Take a few minutes each day to look at your vision board and visualize yourself living that life.
- Say affirmations or prayers while looking at your vision board.
- Feel the emotions of gratitude and excitement as you imagine your dreams coming true.

Remember: Your vision board is a living document. It

can evolve and change as you do. Don't be afraid to add new images, remove old ones, or rearrange the layout. The most important thing is that it continues to inspire and motivate you on your journey towards a purposeful life.

So go ahead, get creative, and let your vision board be a powerful reminder of all that you're capable of achieving!

Day 14: Crafting Your Purpose Statement

Welcome to Day 14! By now, you've delved into the depths of your fears and regrets, started shifting your mindset, and taken some brave steps towards a more empowered you. Today, we're going to take all that incredible work and distill it into something powerful: your very own purpose statement.

Think of your purpose statement as your personal North Star, a guiding light that illuminates your path and keeps you on track. It's a concise declaration of who you are, what you value, and the unique contribution you want to make in the world.

Why is crafting a purpose statement so important? Because it serves as a powerful tool for decision-making, goal setting, and living a life that truly aligns with your values. It's a constant reminder of your "why" – the driving force behind your actions and the source of your motivation.

YOUR PURPOSE STATEMENT AS A COMPASS

Imagine setting off on a cross-country road trip without a

map or GPS. You might wander aimlessly, take wrong turns, or even end up lost and frustrated. The same can happen in life when

we don't have a clear sense of purpose. We may find ourselves drifting from one thing to the next, feeling unfulfilled and unsure of our direction.

A well-crafted purpose statement acts as your compass, providing clarity and direction in the face of uncertainty. It helps you make choices that align with your values and goals, even when faced with tempting distractions or challenging obstacles.

UNLEASHING YOUR POTENTIAL

Your purpose statement isn't just about guiding your actions; it's also about unleashing your full potential. When you have a clear understanding of your "why," you tap into a deeper well of motivation and passion. You become more resilient, more focused, and more determined to create a life that is meaningful and fulfilling.

Think about it: When you're working towards something that truly matters to you, you're more likely to overcome challenges, persevere through setbacks, and achieve your goals. A purpose statement can ignite a fire within you, propelling you towards a life that is truly extraordinary.

CRAFTING YOUR LEGACY

Ultimately, your purpose statement is about crafting your legacy. It's about leaving your mark on the world and creating a life that you'll be proud of. It's about making a positive impact on the lives of others and contributing to something bigger than yourself.

So, are you ready to discover your North Star? In this chapter, we'll guide you through a step-by-step process for crafting a purpose statement that resonates with your heart and soul. We'll explore different approaches, share inspiring examples, and provide you with the tools you need to create a powerful declaration that will guide you towards a life of purpose, passion, and no regrets.

Get ready to uncover the magic that lies within you and embrace the extraordinary life that awaits. Your purpose is calling!

DEFINING YOUR PURPOSE

In the labyrinth of life, it's easy to feel lost, overwhelmed, or uncertain about which path to take. We're bombarded with distractions, obligations, and competing priorities, leaving us questioning our direction and purpose. But what if there was a way to navigate this maze with clarity and confidence? What if you had a personal compass, a guiding light that could illuminate your path and lead you towards a life of greater meaning and fulfillment?

That guiding light is your purpose statement.

Your purpose statement is a clear and concise declaration of your core values, passions, and the unique contribution you want to make in the world. It's a compass that points you in the right direction, a filter for decision-making, and a source of inspiration when challenges arise.

Imagine waking up each morning with a deep sense of knowing *why* you do what you do. Imagine having a clear vision of the impact you want to create, the legacy you want to leave behind. Imagine feeling a sense of purpose that fuels your actions, motivates you through obstacles, and brings a deep sense of fulfillment to your life. That's the power of a well-defined purpose statement.

WHY A PURPOSE STATEMENT MATTERS

A purpose statement is not just a feel-good exercise; it's a practical tool that can transform your life in profound ways. Here's why it matters:

1. **Provides clarity and direction:** A purpose statement helps you identify what truly matters to you, what you're passionate about, and how you want to contribute to the world. This clarity can guide your decisions, both big and small, and help you stay focused on what's most important.
2. **Fuels motivation and resilience:** When you have a clear sense of purpose, you're more likely to persevere through challenges and setbacks. Your purpose becomes a driving force that motivates you to keep going, even when things get tough.
3. **Enhances decision-making:** A purpose statement serves as a filter for evaluating opportunities and choices. When faced with a decision, you can ask yourself, "Does this align with my purpose?" This simple

question can help you make choices that lead you closer to your goals and values.
4. **Increases self-awareness:** Crafting a purpose statement requires deep reflection and self-discovery. It encourages you to explore your values, passions, strengths, and weaknesses, leading to greater self-understanding.
5. **Attracts opportunities:** When you live with purpose, you radiate a certain energy that attracts like-minded people and opportunities. Your passion and commitment become contagious, inspiring others and opening doors you never imagined.

YOUR PURPOSE STATEMENT AS A GUIDING LIGHT

Think of your purpose statement as a North Star, a constant point of reference that guides you on your journey. It's a reminder of what truly matters, a source of inspiration when you feel lost or discouraged, and a touchstone for making choices that align with your authentic self.

It's not about finding the "one perfect purpose" that you're destined to fulfill. Your purpose can evolve and change over time as you grow and learn. The key is to have a clear statement that reflects your current values, passions, and aspirations.

Your purpose statement doesn't have to be grand or complex. It can be a simple sentence or a few words that capture the essence of your "why." What matters most is that it resonates with you and inspires you to take action.

Crafting your purpose statement is a journey of self-discovery. It's about delving deep into your heart and soul, uncovering your passions and values, and identifying the unique

contribution you want to make in the world. It's a process that takes time, reflection, and a willingness to be honest with yourself.

But the rewards are immense. When you have a clear and compelling purpose statement, you'll feel more energized, motivated, and fulfilled. You'll have a sense of direction and purpose that will guide you through life's challenges and lead you towards a life that you love.

PURPOSE STATEMENT EXAMPLES

Imagine a compass guiding you through uncharted territory, a lighthouse illuminating your path on a stormy night, or a North Star keeping you on course even when you feel lost. Your purpose statement can be all of these things and more. It's a powerful declaration that captures the essence of who you are, what you value, and how you want to contribute to the world.

But crafting a purpose statement can feel daunting. Where do you even begin? How do you condense the vastness of your dreams and aspirations into a few concise sentences? To inspire and guide you, let's explore some real-life examples of purpose statements from diverse individuals and professions:

The Entrepreneur: "My purpose is to empower women to achieve financial independence and create businesses that make a positive impact on their communities."

This entrepreneur's purpose statement goes beyond simply

making a profit. It speaks to a deeper desire to uplift others and contribute to a greater cause.

The Artist: "My purpose is to use my art to evoke emotions, spark conversations, and challenge the status quo."

This artist recognizes that their art is not just about aesthetics; it's about making a meaningful impact on the world through creativity and expression.

The Teacher: "My purpose is to inspire a love of learning in my students, to equip them with the skills and knowledge they need to succeed, and to nurture their potential as compassionate and responsible citizens."

This teacher's purpose statement highlights the multiple facets of their role, from imparting knowledge to fostering personal growth and social responsibility.

The Healthcare Professional: "My purpose is to provide compassionate care to my patients, to advocate for their well-being, and to contribute to the advancement of medical knowledge."

This healthcare professional's purpose statement reflects a commitment to patient care, advocacy, and the ongoing pursuit of excellence in their field.

The Environmental Activist: "My purpose is to protect our planet's natural resources, to raise awareness about environmental issues, and to inspire others to take action for a sustainable future."

This activist's purpose statement is a call to action, driven by a deep concern for the environment and a desire to create positive change.

The Parent: "My purpose is to raise children who are

kind, compassionate, and confident, who will make a positive contribution to the world."

This parent's purpose statement emphasizes the importance of nurturing the next generation and instilling values that will shape a better future.

These are just a few examples, but they demonstrate the diversity and power of purpose statements. Notice how they are all:

- **Specific:** They clearly articulate the individual's desired impact or contribution.
- **Actionable:** They focus on verbs and actions, not just lofty ideals.
- **Meaningful:** They connect to the person's values and passions.
- **Inspiring:** They convey a sense of hope, optimism, and possibility.

As you craft your own purpose statement, don't be afraid to experiment and play with different words and phrases. It's a personal declaration, so make it your own. It may evolve and change over time, but it will always serve as a touchstone, reminding you of your "why" and guiding you towards a life of greater fulfillment and impact.

Remember, your purpose statement is not a rigid contract; it's a living document that can adapt and evolve as you do. It's a reminder of your unique gifts and the difference you want to make in the world. So let it guide you, inspire you, and empower you to live a life that's authentically yours.

EXERCISE: PURPOSE STATEMENT DRAFT

Ready to put your purpose into words? Today, we're going to create a first draft of your personal purpose statement. Think of it as your North Star – a guiding light that illuminates your path and keeps you focused on what truly matters.

Don't worry about crafting the perfect statement right away. This is just a starting point, a way to articulate your aspirations and begin to bring them to life.

WHAT IS A PURPOSE STATEMENT?

A purpose statement is a concise declaration that captures the essence of who you are, what you value, and how you want to contribute to the world. It's a personal mantra that can guide your decisions, inspire your actions, and give you a sense of direction.

Your purpose statement doesn't have to be grand or overly ambitious. It can be simple, honest, and heartfelt. It's about what lights you up inside, what drives you, and what you believe your unique contribution can be.

WHY CREATE A PURPOSE STATEMENT?

Having a clear purpose statement can have a profound impact on your life:

- **Clarity and Focus:** It helps you clarify your priorities

and make decisions that align with your values and goals.
- **Motivation and Inspiration:** It fuels your motivation by reminding you of the bigger picture and why your efforts matter.
- **Resilience and Perseverance:** It provides a source of strength during challenging times, reminding you of your "why" and helping you stay on track.
- **Authenticity and Fulfillment:** It encourages you to live a life that is true to yourself and in alignment with your passions and values.

CRAFTING YOUR PURPOSE STATEMENT

Let's get started! Here's a simple framework to help you create your first draft:

1. **Brainstorm Your Verbs:** What actions do you want to take in your life? What do you want to achieve? Think about verbs that resonate with you (e.g., inspire, create, empower, heal, connect, educate, build, transform).
2. **Identify Your Values:** What principles are most important to you? What qualities do you want to embody? Consider values like honesty, compassion, creativity, courage, perseverance, or service.
3. **Define Your Impact:** How do you want to contribute to the world? What difference do you want to make? Think about the positive impact you want to have on others, your community, or the world at large.

Putting It All Together

Now, try combining your verbs, values, and impact words into a single statement. Here are a few examples to get you started:

- "To empower women to embrace their unique voices and create fulfilling lives."
- "To inspire others to live with passion, purpose, and compassion."
- "To use my creativity to foster connection and build community."
- "To lead with integrity, serve with humility, and make a lasting difference in the world."

Your purpose statement can be as long or as short as you like. The most important thing is that it feels authentic and meaningful to you.

Tips for Crafting Your Statement:

- **Keep it concise:** Aim for a statement that is memorable and easy to repeat.
- **Use strong verbs:** Verbs convey action and energy. Choose verbs that inspire and motivate you.
- **Incorporate your values:** Your purpose statement should reflect the principles that are most important to you.
- **Focus on impact:** How do you want to make a difference? Your purpose statement should highlight your unique contribution.
- **Make it personal:** This is *your* purpose statement.

Don't worry about what others might think or say. Make it yours.

Don't Overthink It!

Remember, this is just a first draft. Your purpose statement can evolve and change over time as you learn and grow. The most important thing is to start somewhere.

Don't get caught up in trying to create the perfect statement. Just start writing. Let your thoughts flow freely and see what emerges. You might be surprised by what you discover.

Next Steps:

Once you've crafted your initial purpose statement, take some time to reflect on it. Does it resonate with you? Does it feel authentic and true to who you are? If not, don't worry. You can always revise and refine it later.

Share your purpose statement with a trusted friend, family member, or mentor. Ask for their feedback and see if they have any insights or suggestions.

Most importantly, keep your purpose statement visible. Write it down, put it on your vision board, or set it as a reminder on your phone. Let it serve as a constant reminder of your "why" and inspire you to live each day with intention.

This is just the beginning of your journey towards living a purposeful life. Embrace it, explore it, and watch as your purpose unfolds before you.

Day 15: Power Poses

Ever feel like you're shrinking into yourself, your shoulders hunched, your gaze lowered? Maybe it's before a big presentation, a tough conversation, or even just facing a new day. It's as if our bodies mirror our doubts and anxieties, reinforcing a cycle of insecurity.

But what if I told you that you could actually reverse this? What if simply changing your posture for a few minutes could ignite a spark of confidence within you?

Welcome to the world of power poses.

It might sound a bit unusual, but research has shown that the way we hold our bodies can significantly impact our minds and emotions. It's a two-way street: our thoughts and feelings influence our posture, and our posture, in turn, influences our thoughts and feelings.

So, if we consciously adopt poses that exude confidence and power, even when we don't necessarily feel that way on the inside, we can actually trick our brains into feeling more self-assured. It's like a shortcut to feeling empowered, even when faced with challenges or self-doubt.

Think of it this way: our bodies are not just vessels for our minds; they are active participants in our emotional and mental states. When we stand tall, shoulders back, head held high, we signal to ourselves that we are capable, strong, and worthy. This physical display of confidence triggers a cascade of biochemical reactions in our brains, increasing testosterone (the hormone associated with dominance and power) and decreasing cortisol (the stress hormone).

In this chapter, we're going to dive into the fascinating world of power poses and explore how you can use them to boost your confidence, reduce stress, and step into your personal power. You'll learn about the science behind these poses, discover simple yet effective poses you can practice, and get tips on how to integrate them into your daily life.

So, are you ready to stand tall, own your space, and radiate confidence? Get ready to unleash your inner superhero with the power of posture!

THE MIND-BODY CONNECTION

Have you ever noticed how your body language changes depending on your mood? When you're feeling confident, you stand tall, shoulders back, head held high. When you're feeling defeated, you slump, cross your arms, and avoid eye contact. This isn't just a coincidence; it's a direct reflection of the powerful mind-body connection.

Our bodies and minds are not separate entities; they are intimately intertwined. Our thoughts and emotions influence our physical sensations, and our physical sensations, in turn, affect our thoughts and emotions. This mind-body loop is a constant feedback system, with each influencing the other.

Think about it: When you're anxious, your heart might

race, your palms sweat, and your stomach churns. Conversely, when you're feeling joyful, you might smile, laugh, and feel a lightness in your step. Our bodies are constantly communicating with our minds, sending signals that shape our emotions and perceptions.

So, what does this mean for you? It means that you have more control over your emotions and thoughts than you might realize. By consciously shifting your body language, you can actually change the way you feel. This is where the fascinating concept of power posing comes in.

THE SCIENCE BEHIND POWER POSING

Power posing, popularized by social psychologist Amy Cuddy, refers to adopting expansive and open body postures that convey confidence and power. Think of a superhero standing with their hands on their hips, chest out, and chin up. These postures, even held for a short period, have been shown to have a profound impact on our hormones and neurotransmitters.

Research suggests that power posing can increase levels of testosterone (associated with confidence and assertiveness) and decrease levels of cortisol (the stress hormone). This hormonal shift can lead to feelings of greater confidence, reduced anxiety, and improved performance in stressful situations.

But it's not just about the hormones. Power posing also affects our thoughts and perceptions. When we stand tall and open, we literally take up more space, which can make us feel more powerful and in control. This shift in perception can lead to more positive self-talk, increased optimism, and a greater willingness to take risks.

PUTTING POWER POSING INTO PRACTICE

Now that you understand the science behind power posing, you might be wondering how to incorporate it into your daily life. Here are a few simple steps:

1. **Choose Your Pose:** There are several effective power poses. Some popular ones include:
    - **The Wonder Woman Pose:** Stand with your feet shoulder-width apart, hands on hips, chest lifted and chin up.
    - **The Victory Pose:** Raise your arms in a V shape above your head, like you just won a race.
    - **The CEO Pose:** Lean back in your chair with your arms behind your head, legs crossed, and a relaxed expression.
2. **Hold the Pose:** Hold your chosen pose for 2-3 minutes. Close your eyes if it helps you focus. Breathe deeply and notice any sensations in your body.
3. **Repeat Regularly:** Practice power posing daily, ideally before a stressful situation like a job interview, presentation, or important conversation.

REAL-LIFE APPLICATIONS

Power posing isn't just for superheroes. It's a practical tool you can use to boost your confidence and performance in various situations. Here are a few examples:

- **Job Interviews:** Before entering the interview room, take a few minutes to strike a power pose in the restroom or a private space.
- **Presentations:** Stand in a power pose before taking the stage to calm your nerves and project confidence.
- **Networking Events:** Use open body language and power poses to make a strong first impression.
- **Difficult Conversations:** Hold a power pose before a challenging conversation to feel more assertive and in control.

Remember, power posing isn't about faking confidence; it's about tapping into your inner strength and projecting it outward. It's a simple yet effective tool that can help you overcome self-doubt, manage stress, and achieve your goals.

PRACTICING POWER POSES

Okay, friend, let's get physical! No, we're not hitting the gym (although that's always a good idea for your overall well-being!). We're going to channel our inner superheroes and practice some power poses.

You might be wondering, "What do power poses have to do with living a regret-free life?" Well, it turns out that our body language isn't just a reflection of how we feel; it can actually influence our emotions and thoughts. When we stand tall, open up our posture, and take up space, it sends signals to our brains that we are confident, powerful, and capable. And guess what? Our brains believe it!

THE SCIENCE BEHIND POWER POSES

Research has shown that power posing for just two minutes can significantly increase testosterone (the dominance hormone) and decrease cortisol (the stress hormone) in our bodies. This hormonal shift leads to increased feelings of confidence, decreased anxiety, and a greater willingness to take risks.

So, even if you don't *feel* confident, striking a power pose can trick your brain into believing that you are. It's like putting on a superhero cape – even though it's just a piece of fabric, it can make you feel invincible.

POWER POSES FOR EVERYDAY CONFIDENCE

Let's explore a few simple power poses that you can practice anywhere, anytime:

1. **The Wonder Woman Pose:** Stand with your feet shoulder-width apart, hands on your hips, chin lifted, and chest open. Imagine yourself as Wonder Woman, ready to take on the world. Hold this pose for two minutes, breathing deeply and feeling your power expand.
2. **The Victory Pose:** Stand tall with your arms raised in a V-shape above your head. Picture yourself crossing a finish line or achieving a major goal. Hold this pose

for two minutes, feeling the rush of accomplishment and pride.
3. **The CEO Pose:** Sit in a chair with your back straight, hands behind your head, fingers interlaced. Lean back slightly, projecting openness and confidence. Imagine yourself leading a successful business meeting or making a major decision. Hold this pose for two minutes, feeling a sense of authority and control.
4. **The Loomer Pose:** This one's my personal favorite! Stand tall with your feet hip-width apart and your hands loosely clasped behind your back. Lean forward slightly from your hips, keeping your back straight and your head held high. Imagine yourself towering over a challenge, ready to tackle it head-on. Hold this pose for two minutes, feeling your confidence and determination soar.

TIPS FOR MAXIMUM EFFECT

Here are a few tips to make the most of your power posing practice:

- **Privacy:** If you're not comfortable striking a pose in public, find a private space where you can let loose. Your bathroom, bedroom, or even a quiet corner of the office can work.
- **Music:** Put on some upbeat music that makes you feel empowered and confident.
- **Visualization:** While holding the pose, visualize your-

self achieving your goals and dreams. See yourself as the confident, successful person you aspire to be.
- **Affirmations:** Repeat positive affirmations that align with the pose. For example, while holding the Wonder Woman pose, you might say, "I am strong, capable, and unstoppable."

POWER POSING IN REAL LIFE

You don't have to limit your power posing to designated practice sessions. You can incorporate it into your everyday life:

- **Before a job interview:** Strike a power pose in the restroom to boost your confidence.
- **Before a presentation:** Channel your inner CEO with a power pose in your office.
- **When feeling stressed:** Take a few minutes to practice the Wonder Woman pose or the Victory pose.
- **Anytime you need a confidence boost:** Remember, you have a superhero within you!

By practicing power poses regularly, you'll rewire your brain to associate those postures with feelings of confidence, power, and success. This can have a profound impact on your mindset, your behavior, and ultimately, your ability to live a regret-free life.

EXERCISE: POWER POSES

Okay, friend, it's time to unleash your inner superhero! Today's exercise involves a bit of playfulness and might even make you feel a little silly at first. But trust me, the benefits are worth it. We're going to practice power poses – specific postures that have been scientifically proven to boost confidence, reduce stress hormones, and increase feelings of power.

Think about your favorite superhero for a moment. How do they stand? Tall, expansive, with their shoulders back and head held high? They exude confidence and power, ready to take on any challenge. You might be surprised to learn that simply by changing your posture, you can tap into those same feelings.

Here's the science behind it: When we hold our bodies in expansive, powerful postures, it triggers a cascade of hormonal changes. Our levels of testosterone (the dominance hormone) rise, while cortisol (the stress hormone) decreases. This shift in our biochemistry leads to increased confidence, optimism, and a greater sense of personal power.

THE POWER POSE PRACTICE

1. **The Wonder Woman:** Stand with your feet shoulder-width apart, hands on your hips, chin lifted, and chest open. Imagine you're ready to take on the world. Hold this pose for 2 minutes, breathing deeply and feeling your strength.
2. **The Victory Pose:** Raise your arms overhead in a V-shape, as if you've just won a race or achieved a major

goal. Feel the energy coursing through your body as you hold this triumphant pose for 2 minutes.

3. **The CEO:** Sit down with your legs crossed and lean back in your chair, hands clasped behind your head. This is the pose of a confident leader, surveying their domain. Hold it for 2 minutes, breathing deeply and feeling a sense of calm authority.

You can experiment with other power poses as well. The key is to choose postures that make you feel strong, confident, and in control.

NOTICE THE SHIFT

As you practice these power poses, pay attention to your body and your emotions. Notice any shifts in your mood, energy levels, or thoughts. Do you feel more confident? More relaxed? More optimistic?

Don't worry if you don't feel a dramatic shift right away. The effects of power posing can be subtle at first. But with consistent practice, you'll start to notice a difference in how you carry yourself, how you interact with others, and how you approach challenges.

INTEGRATE POWER POSES INTO YOUR LIFE

You don't have to limit your power posing to this exercise. You can incorporate it into your daily routine. Try standing in a power pose before a big meeting or presentation. Strike a victory pose after completing a challenging task. Or simply take a few minutes each day to stand tall and expansive, reminding yourself of your inner strength and resilience.

Remember, power posing is not about pretending to be someone you're not. It's about tapping into your inherent power and confidence. It's about reminding yourself that you are capable, strong, and worthy of success.

YOUR SUPERHERO WITHIN

So go ahead, embrace your inner superhero! Stand tall, open your heart, and claim your power. By simply changing your posture, you can change your mindset and create a more positive, empowering reality.

As you continue to practice power posing, you'll find yourself feeling more confident, more resilient, and more ready to take on whatever life throws your way. You'll tap into a wellspring of inner strength that you may not have even known existed. And that, my friend, is the true power of living with intention.

Day 16: Review and Refine Purpose Statement

Remember that exhilarating feeling when you first put pen to paper and started drafting your purpose statement? It was a moment of clarity, a glimpse into the heart of what truly drives you.

But, like a rough diamond, your initial statement may need some polishing to truly sparkle. That's why today is all about refining your purpose statement, turning it into a beacon that guides your every decision and action.

Think of your purpose statement as your personal compass. It points you in the right direction, helping you navigate life's twists and turns with confidence and clarity. A well-crafted purpose statement becomes your North Star, reminding you of your "why" and keeping you on track towards a life of fulfillment.

But what exactly makes a good purpose statement? It's not just a catchy slogan or a list of goals. It's a concise, powerful declaration that captures the essence of who you are, what you value, and how you want to contribute to the world.

A strong purpose statement is:

- **Meaningful:** It speaks to your heart and soul, aligning with your deepest values and aspirations.
- **Actionable:** It provides a clear direction for your actions and decisions, helping you stay focused on what truly matters.
- **Inspiring:** It motivates you to get out of bed each morning, excited to pursue your goals and dreams.
- **Authentic:** It reflects your unique personality, talents, and passions.

Today, we'll revisit your initial draft, refine it, and ensure it meets these criteria. We'll also explore the power of sharing your purpose statement with others, as this can create accountability, inspire those around you, and open up new opportunities.

This is a process of self-discovery and refinement. Don't be afraid to experiment, try different wording, and see what resonates most deeply with you. Remember, your purpose statement isn't set in stone; it can evolve and change as you grow and evolve.

The goal is to create a statement that not only guides your actions but also fills you with a sense of excitement and purpose. It should be something you're proud to share with the world, a testament to the unique value you bring to the table.

So, grab your journal, your favorite pen, and let's dive

into the process of refining your purpose statement. This is your chance

to sharpen your compass, set your course, and embark on a journey toward a life that truly lights you up.

REFINE YOUR DRAFT

Remember that purpose statement you drafted a few days ago? It's time to dust it off, give it a fresh look, and see if it still resonates with the person you are now.

Think of your purpose statement like a compass. It helps you navigate life's twists and turns, guiding you towards decisions and actions that align with your true north. But just like a compass needs to be adjusted occasionally to stay accurate, your purpose statement might need some fine-tuning as you evolve and grow.

The past few weeks have been a journey of self-discovery. You've dug deep into your fears, regrets, values, and passions. You've explored your strengths, clarified your vision, and started taking purposeful action. All of these experiences have likely shifted your perspective and deepened your understanding of yourself.

As a result, your initial purpose statement might not fully capture the essence of who you are and what you want to achieve. It might feel too broad, too narrow, or simply not quite right. That's perfectly okay! Your purpose is not set in stone; it's a living, breathing entity that evolves alongside you.

So, How Do You Refine Your Purpose Statement?

Here are a few questions to guide your reflection:

1. **Does it feel authentic?** Does your purpose statement genuinely reflect your values, passions, and aspirations? Does it resonate with your heart and soul?
2. **Is it clear and concise?** Can you easily explain your purpose to someone else? Does it capture the essence of what you want to achieve in a few sentences?
3. **Is it actionable?** Does your purpose statement inspire you to take action? Does it give you a clear sense of direction and purpose in your daily life?
4. **Is it adaptable?** Can your purpose statement evolve and grow with you as you change and experience new things?

If your answer to any of these questions is "no," then it's time to refine your purpose statement.

Here are some tips for refining your purpose statement:

- **Review your "What If" inventory:** Are there any recurring themes or patterns that point to a deeper purpose?
- **Reflect on your values assessment:** Do your core values shine through in your purpose statement?
- **Consider your passions and strengths:** How can you use your unique gifts to make a difference in the world?
- **Look at your vision board:** Does your purpose statement align with the images and words that represent your dreams?
- **Seek feedback from others:** Ask a trusted friend, family member, or mentor for their honest opinion of your purpose statement.

Remember, there is no right or wrong way to write a purpose statement. The most important thing is that it feels true and meaningful to you. It should be a source of inspiration, motivation, and guidance as you navigate your life's journey.

THE EVOLUTION OF PURPOSE

Your purpose statement is not a destination; it's a starting point. As you grow and change, your purpose will evolve alongside you. It's okay to revisit and refine your purpose statement periodically as you gain new experiences, insights, and perspectives.

Embrace the evolution of your purpose. It's a sign that you're growing, learning, and expanding your horizons. Your purpose is not meant to be static; it's a dynamic force that fuels your passion, ignites your creativity, and guides you towards a life of meaning and fulfillment.

So, take some time to reflect on your purpose statement. Revise it, refine it, and make it your own. Let it be a reflection of who you are, what you value, and what you want to contribute to the world. And remember, this is just the beginning. Your purpose is waiting to be lived.

SHARING YOUR PURPOSE

You've done the deep work. You've unearthed your passions, faced your fears, and crafted a purpose statement that resonates with your soul. Now, it's time to unleash that purpose into the world. But here's the thing: purpose isn't meant to be kept hidden away like a secret treasure. It's meant to be shared.

WHY SHARE YOUR PURPOSE?

You might be wondering, "Why should I share my purpose with others? Isn't it personal?" Absolutely! But sharing your purpose is not about seeking validation or approval. It's about amplifying your impact, creating a ripple effect that extends far beyond yourself.

Here's why sharing your purpose can be a game-changer:

1. **Accountability:** When you share your purpose with others, you create a sense of accountability. You're not just making a promise to yourself; you're making a declaration to the world. This can be incredibly motivating, as it encourages you to stay committed to your goals and take action even when things get tough.
2. **Support and Connection:** Sharing your purpose opens the door to support and connection. When others know what you're working towards, they can offer encouragement, guidance, and resources. They can become your cheerleaders, mentors, and collaborators, helping you stay on track and overcome obstacles.
3. **Inspiration:** Your purpose has the power to inspire others. When you share your story and your passion, you may spark a flame in someone else, encouraging them to pursue their own dreams and make a difference in the world.
4. **Opportunities:** Sharing your purpose can open up

unexpected doors and opportunities. You may find yourself connecting with like-minded individuals, landing your dream job, or even creating a movement that changes the world.

5. **Clarity and Focus:** Articulating your purpose to others forces you to clarify your own thoughts and priorities. It helps you solidify your vision and stay focused on what truly matters.
6. **Legacy:** By sharing your purpose, you're not just living for today; you're creating a legacy that will outlive you. You're inspiring future generations to live with intention, passion, and a commitment to making a positive impact.

HOW TO SHARE YOUR PURPOSE

Sharing your purpose doesn't have to be a grand gesture. It can be as simple as:

- **Talking to loved ones:** Share your purpose statement with your family, friends, or partner. Tell them what you're working towards and why it's important to you.
- **Networking:** Connect with people in your field or industry who share your passion. Attend conferences, workshops, or online events where you can share your ideas and goals.
- **Social media:** Use social media platforms to share your story, your passion, and your progress. Engage with others who are on a similar path and build a community of support.

- **Creating content:** Start a blog, podcast, or YouTube channel where you can share your expertise and inspire others.
- **Volunteering or mentoring:** Use your talents and skills to serve others. Volunteer your time, mentor someone who is just starting out, or find ways to give back to your community.

OVERCOMING THE FEAR OF SHARING

Sharing your purpose can be intimidating. You might worry about judgment, criticism, or even failure. But remember, vulnerability is a strength, not a weakness. When you share your authentic self with the world, you open yourself up to deeper connections, greater opportunities, and a more fulfilling life.

Here are a few tips for overcoming the fear of sharing your purpose:

- **Start small:** You don't have to share your purpose with the entire world right away. Begin by sharing it with people you trust and who you know will support you.
- **Focus on your passion:** Don't get caught up in trying to be perfect or having all the answers. Share your passion and enthusiasm for your purpose, and let that shine through.
- **Find your tribe:** Seek out communities of like-minded individuals who will understand and support your journey.
- **Embrace vulnerability:** Don't be afraid to show your

human side. Share your challenges, setbacks, and lessons learned. This will make you more relatable and inspiring to others.
- **Remember your "why":** When you feel hesitant, remind yourself of why you're doing this. Connect to your deeper purpose and the impact you want to make in the world.

YOUR PURPOSE IS A GIFT

Your purpose is a gift, not just to you, but to the world. By sharing it, you're not only living a more authentic and fulfilling life, but you're also contributing to something bigger than yourself. You're leaving a legacy, inspiring others, and making a positive impact on the world. So don't be afraid to let your light shine.

Share your purpose with courage, passion, and authenticity. The world is waiting for you.

EXERCISE: SHARE YOUR PURPOSE STATEMENT

You've done the hard work of crafting a purpose statement that reflects your values, passions, and unique gifts. It's a powerful declaration of who you are and what you want to contribute to the world. But now, it's time to take a brave step and share your purpose statement with someone you trust.

Why Share?

Sharing your purpose statement might feel vulnerable, but it's a crucial step on your journey to living a regret-free life. Here's why:

1. **Accountability:** When you share your purpose with someone else, you create a sense of accountability. Knowing that someone else is aware of your intentions can help you stay motivated and on track.
2. **Clarity:** Sharing your purpose out loud can help you gain even greater clarity about your goals and aspirations. As you explain your purpose to someone else, you might discover new nuances or insights that you hadn't considered before.
3. **Support:** A trusted friend, family member, or mentor can offer invaluable support and encouragement as you pursue your purpose. They can celebrate your wins, offer guidance during challenges, and help you stay focused on your path.
4. **Feedback:** Getting feedback on your purpose statement can help you refine it further. Perhaps there are aspects of your statement that aren't clear or that could be worded more powerfully. The insights of others can help you create a purpose statement that truly resonates with you.
5. **Inspiration:** Sharing your purpose can inspire others to do the same. You might be surprised by how your vulnerability and openness can empower others to discover their own passions and goals.

CHOOSING YOUR CONFIDANTE

Who should you share your purpose statement with? Choose
someone who you trust implicitly, someone who believes in you and wants to see you succeed. It could be:

- **A close friend:** Someone who knows you well and who you can have open and honest conversations with.
- **A family member:** A parent, sibling, or other relative who supports your dreams and aspirations.
- **A mentor:** Someone you look up to and who has experience in a field or area of life that you're interested in.
- **A coach or therapist:** A professional who can offer unbiased feedback and support.

PREPARING FOR THE CONVERSATION

Before sharing your purpose statement, take some time to reflect on the following:

- **What are you hoping to gain from this conversation?** Clarity? Support? Feedback? Knowing your intentions will help you guide the conversation.
- **How do you want to feel after sharing your purpose statement?** Empowered? Confident? Motivated? Setting an intention for the conversation can help you manifest those feelings.
- **What are your concerns or hesitations?** Are you worried about judgment or criticism? Addressing your

Sharing your purpose statement might feel vulnerable, but it's a crucial step on your journey to living a regret-free life. Here's why:

1. **Accountability:** When you share your purpose with someone else, you create a sense of accountability. Knowing that someone else is aware of your intentions can help you stay motivated and on track.
2. **Clarity:** Sharing your purpose out loud can help you gain even greater clarity about your goals and aspirations. As you explain your purpose to someone else, you might discover new nuances or insights that you hadn't considered before.
3. **Support:** A trusted friend, family member, or mentor can offer invaluable support and encouragement as you pursue your purpose. They can celebrate your wins, offer guidance during challenges, and help you stay focused on your path.
4. **Feedback:** Getting feedback on your purpose statement can help you refine it further. Perhaps there are aspects of your statement that aren't clear or that could be worded more powerfully. The insights of others can help you create a purpose statement that truly resonates with you.
5. **Inspiration:** Sharing your purpose can inspire others to do the same. You might be surprised by how your vulnerability and openness can empower others to discover their own passions and goals.

CHOOSING YOUR CONFIDANTE

Who should you share your purpose statement with? Choose
someone who you trust implicitly, someone who believes in you and wants to see you succeed. It could be:

- **A close friend:** Someone who knows you well and who you can have open and honest conversations with.
- **A family member:** A parent, sibling, or other relative who supports your dreams and aspirations.
- **A mentor:** Someone you look up to and who has experience in a field or area of life that you're interested in.
- **A coach or therapist:** A professional who can offer unbiased feedback and support.

PREPARING FOR THE CONVERSATION

Before sharing your purpose statement, take some time to reflect on the following:

- **What are you hoping to gain from this conversation?** Clarity? Support? Feedback? Knowing your intentions will help you guide the conversation.
- **How do you want to feel after sharing your purpose statement?** Empowered? Confident? Motivated? Setting an intention for the conversation can help you manifest those feelings.
- **What are your concerns or hesitations?** Are you worried about judgment or criticism? Addressing your

concerns beforehand can help you approach the conversation with more confidence.

SHARING YOUR PURPOSE STATEMENT

When you're ready to share your purpose statement, find a quiet, comfortable space where you won't be interrupted. Start by explaining why you're sharing this with them and what you hope to gain from the conversation. Then, read your purpose statement aloud.

As they listen, pay attention to their body language and facial expressions. Do they seem engaged and supportive? Are they asking thoughtful questions? After you've finished reading your purpose statement, invite their feedback. Ask them what stands out to them, what resonates with them, and if they have any suggestions for improvement.

Remember, this is a dialogue, not a monologue. Be open to their feedback, even if it's not what you expected. Use their insights to refine your purpose statement and make it even more powerful.

BEYOND SHARING

Once you've shared your purpose statement with your confidante, don't let it gather dust. Keep it somewhere visible as a daily reminder of your goals and aspirations. Refer to it often as you make decisions, set priorities, and navigate life's challenges.

Consider sharing your purpose statement with others as well. It could be a post on social media, a conversation with a colleague, or even a presentation at a conference. The more you share your purpose, the more it will become ingrained in your life and the more you'll attract opportunities that align with your goals.

Remember, your purpose is a gift to the world. By sharing it with others, you not only empower yourself but also inspire others to live their lives with intention and purpose. So don't be afraid to let your light shine, my friend. The world needs your unique gifts.

Day 17: Continue Self-Talk Audit/ Reframing

Remember that little voice inside your head? The one that whispers (or sometimes shouts!) commentary on everything you do, think, and feel? That's your self-talk. And just like any conversation, it can be supportive and uplifting or critical and discouraging.

By now, you've spent some time listening in on this inner dialogue through your self-talk audit. Perhaps you've noticed patterns – recurring themes of self-doubt, worry, or criticism that tend to pop up in certain situations. Maybe you've even caught yourself saying things you wouldn't dream of saying to a friend.

Don't worry, you're not alone. We all have an inner critic. It's part of being human. But the good news is that you have the power to change the conversation. You can learn to challenge those negative thoughts, reframe them into more positive ones, and ultimately, create a more supportive and empowering inner dialogue.

Why does this matter? Because your self-talk has a direct impact on your emotions, behaviors, and overall well-being. If you constantly tell yourself you're not good enough, you'll start to believe it. If you focus on your flaws and mistakes, you'll miss out on your strengths and accomplishments. But if you cultivate a positive and encouraging inner voice, you'll build confidence, resilience, and a greater sense of self-worth.

This isn't about denying challenges or pretending everything is perfect. It's about recognizing that your thoughts are not facts. They are interpretations, perspectives, and often, they are distorted by fear, insecurity, or past experiences.

By practicing self-talk awareness and reframing, you can:

- **Reduce stress and anxiety:** Negative self-talk fuels stress and worry. By challenging those thoughts, you can create a calmer, more peaceful mind.
- **Boost confidence and self-esteem:** Affirming your strengths and capabilities can help you feel more confident and capable.
- **Improve your relationships:** When you treat yourself with kindness and respect, you're more likely to attract positive and supportive relationships.
- **Increase motivation and resilience:** A positive inner dialogue can help you overcome setbacks, bounce back from challenges, and stay focused on your goals.
- **Achieve your dreams:** When you believe in yourself, you're more likely to take risks, pursue your passions, and create a life that you love.

So how do you do it? How do you change a lifelong

habit of negative self-talk? It takes time, effort, and practice. But it's absolutely possible. And today, we're going to take another step in that direction. We'll dive deeper into identifying patterns in your self-talk and explore even more powerful techniques for reframing those negative thoughts.

Remember, this is a journey, not a destination. There will be setbacks and challenges along the way. But with patience, persistence, and a willingness to change the conversation within, you can create a more positive, empowering, and supportive inner voice that will propel you towards a regret-free life.

IDENTIFYING PATTERNS

By now, you've spent some time eavesdropping on your inner dialogue, jotting down those sneaky negative thoughts that creep in throughout your day. It might feel a bit like you've been spying on yourself, but trust me, this self-awareness is a game-changer.

Think of your self-talk audit as a treasure map – a map that leads you straight to the heart of your limiting beliefs and fears. It reveals the patterns that have been holding you back, often without you even realizing it. Now, it's time to decipher those patterns and understand the root causes behind them.

UNRAVELING THE TAPESTRY OF YOUR THOUGHTS

As you review your self-talk audit, you may notice some recurring themes. Perhaps you tend to criticize yourself harshly when facing a challenge, or maybe you doubt your abilities

when stepping into new territory. You might find that certain situations or interactions trigger a cascade of negative thoughts.

These patterns aren't random; they're often deeply ingrained in our subconscious, shaped by past experiences, societal messages, and even our own biology. By identifying these patterns, you can start to unravel the tangled threads of your thoughts and gain a deeper understanding of why you think and feel the way you do.

COMMON NEGATIVE SELF-TALK PATTERNS:

- **The Perfectionist:** "I'm not good enough unless everything is perfect."
- **The Catastrophizer:** "This is going to be a disaster. I'm going to mess it up."
- **The Mind Reader:** "They probably think I'm stupid/incompetent/unworthy."
- **The Blamer:** "It's all my fault. I should have known better."
- **The Pessimist:** "Nothing ever goes right for me. Why even bother trying?"

These are just a few examples, and your own patterns may be different. The key is to be open and honest with yourself as you examine your self-talk. Don't judge yourself for having negative thoughts; everyone has them. The goal is simply to become aware of them so you can start to challenge and change them.

UNCOVERING THE ROOTS OF YOUR NEGATIVE SELF-TALK

Once you've identified your patterns, it's time to dig deeper and
explore the root causes. This is where the real transformation happens.

Ask yourself these questions:

- **Where did these negative beliefs come from?** Were they instilled by critical parents, teachers, or peers? Did they stem from past failures or traumatic experiences?
- **What situations or people trigger these thoughts?** Are there specific environments or individuals that tend to bring out your inner critic?
- **What are the underlying fears driving these thoughts?** Are you afraid of failure, rejection, not being good enough, or something else?
- **What are the consequences of these negative thoughts?** How do they affect your behavior, decisions, and relationships?

Answering these questions can be challenging, but it's essential for breaking free from the grip of negative self-talk. Once you understand the origins of your thoughts, you can start to challenge their validity and replace them with more positive and empowering beliefs.

SEEKING SUPPORT ON YOUR JOURNEY

If you find it difficult to identify patterns or uncover the root causes of your negative self-talk, don't hesitate to seek support. A therapist, counselor, or coach can provide guidance and tools for exploring these deeper issues. Remember, there's no shame in asking for help. In fact, it's a sign of strength and courage.

As you continue to explore your self-talk patterns, be patient

and kind to yourself. This process takes time and effort, but the rewards are well worth it. By understanding the roots of your negative thoughts, you'll gain the power to challenge them, reframe them, and ultimately transform your inner dialogue.

In the next section, we'll delve into specific strategies for strengthening your positive self-talk and silencing your inner critic. Get ready to step into a new chapter of self-belief, empowerment, and intentional living.

STRENGTHENING POSITIVE SELF-TALK

Remember that little voice inside your head? The one that sometimes whispers doubts, criticisms, and negativity? We all have it. It's like a constant companion, chattering away in the background of our lives. But what if we could turn that voice into our biggest cheerleader, our most supportive friend? That's the power of positive self-talk.

You've already started practicing affirmations, which is a fantastic first step. Now, let's dive deeper into how you can cultivate a more positive inner dialogue that fuels your confidence, resilience, and overall well-being.

REPLACE SELF-CRITICISM WITH SELF-COMPASSION

We're often our own harshest critics. We beat ourselves up for mistakes, shortcomings, and perceived failures. This negative self-talk can erode our self-esteem and keep us stuck in a cycle of self-doubt. It's time to break free from this habit and replace self-criticism with self-compassion.

Think of how you would talk to a friend who's going through a tough time. You wouldn't berate them or call them names, would you? You'd offer kindness, understanding, and support. Extend that same compassion to yourself. Acknowledge your struggles, forgive your mistakes, and remind yourself that you're human, and that everyone makes mistakes.

Instead of saying, "I'm so stupid for messing that up," try saying, "I made a mistake, but that's okay. I'm learning and growing." Instead of "I'll never be good enough," say, "I'm doing my best, and that's all I can ask of myself." Notice how this shift in language feels. It's a small change, but it can have a profound impact on your mindset and well-being.

FOCUS ON SOLUTIONS, NOT PROBLEMS

It's easy to get caught up in problems and dwell on what's going wrong. But this negativity only amplifies our stress and makes it harder to find a way out. When challenges arise, try shifting your focus from the problem to the solution. Ask yourself empowering questions like:

- "What can I learn from this situation?"
- "What steps can I take to move forward?"
- "What resources or support do I need to overcome this challenge?"

By focusing on solutions, you activate your problem-solving skills and empower yourself to take action. You shift from feeling helpless and overwhelmed to feeling capable and resourceful.

HARNESS THE POWER OF AFFIRMATIONS

You've already started practicing affirmations, and I encourage you to continue. Choose affirmations that resonate with you and address the specific areas where you need support. Write them down, say them out loud, and even post them in places where you'll see them regularly.

Here are a few examples of affirmations you can use:

- "I am capable of achieving my goals."
- "I am worthy of love and happiness."
- "I am strong, resilient, and resourceful."
- "I trust my intuition and make wise choices."
- "I am grateful for all the blessings in my life."

Repeating these affirmations with conviction can help

rewire your brain for positivity and self-belief. Remember, the more you say them, the more you'll believe them.

CHALLENGE NEGATIVE THOUGHTS

When negative thoughts pop up, don't just accept them as truth. Challenge them with evidence. Ask yourself:

- "Is this thought really true?"
- "What evidence do I have to support this thought?"
- "Is there another way to look at this situation?"

Often, you'll find that your negative thoughts are based on fear or insecurity, not reality. By challenging them, you can break their power and create space for more positive and empowering thoughts.

SURROUND YOURSELF WITH POSITIVITY

The people we spend time with have a significant impact on our thoughts and feelings. If you're constantly surrounded by negativity, it's hard to maintain a positive outlook. Seek out supportive friends, family members, or mentors who uplift you and encourage your dreams. Limit your exposure to negative news and social media. Fill your life with books, podcasts, and activities that inspire and motivate you.

CELEBRATE YOUR WINS

Don't wait until you achieve a major goal to celebrate.

Acknowledge and appreciate your small victories along the way. This could be completing a task, learning a new skill, or simply having a positive interaction. Celebrating your wins reinforces positive behavior and builds momentum towards your larger goals.

BE PATIENT WITH YOURSELF

Changing your self-talk takes time and practice. There will be days when you slip back into old patterns. Don't beat yourself up about it. Just acknowledge it, forgive yourself, and recommit to your positive self-talk practice.

By consistently applying these strategies, you'll cultivate a more positive inner dialogue that supports your goals, empowers your choices, and helps you live a life of purpose, passion, and no regrets. Remember, your thoughts are powerful. Choose them wisely.

EXERCISE: REFRAMING CHALLENGE

Now that you've honed your skills in identifying negative self-

talk and practicing affirmations, it's time to apply these tools to a real-life challenge. This exercise will help you reframe a current or anticipated difficulty, transforming your perspective and empowering you to approach it with more confidence and optimism.

Step 1: Identify Your Challenge Think about a situation in your life that's causing you stress, anxiety, or worry. It could be a work project, a relationship issue, a health concern, or any other challenge you're facing. Write it down in a few sentences, describing the situation as objectively as possible.

Step 2: Uncover Your Underlying Thoughts Now, dig deeper into your thoughts and feelings about this challenge. What are the specific worries, doubts, or negative self-talk that come up when you think about it? Write down these thoughts as honestly as you can. Don't worry about being judgmental; just get them out on paper.

Step 3: Challenge Your Thoughts Examine each of these thoughts critically. Are they based on facts or assumptions? Are they helpful or unhelpful? Are they empowering or disempowering? Challenge the validity of each thought by asking yourself questions like:

- *Is this thought 100% true?*
- *What evidence do I have to support this thought?*
- *What evidence do I have to refute this thought?*
- *Is this thought helping me or hurting me?*
- *What would a more positive and empowering thought look like?*

Step 4: Reframe Your Thoughts For each negative thought, create a positive reframe. This doesn't mean ignoring the challenge or pretending everything is perfect. It's about shifting your perspective to a more optimistic and solution-oriented one. Here are some examples:

- **Original Thought:** "I'm going to fail this presentation."

- **Reframed Thought:** "I am well-prepared and capable of delivering a great presentation."
- **Original Thought:** "I'm never going to find love."
- **Reframed Thought:** "I am open to love and deserving of a healthy, fulfilling relationship."
- **Original Thought:** "This situation is hopeless."
- **Reframed Thought:** "This situation is challenging, but I can find solutions and learn from this experience."

Step 5: Practice Your Reframes Repeat your reframed thoughts to yourself regularly. Write them down, say them out loud, or even create visual reminders (like sticky notes or phone wallpapers) to reinforce them. The more you practice these new, positive thoughts, the more natural they will become, and the more they will influence your emotions and actions.

Step 6: Take Action With a more positive and empowered mindset, start taking action towards addressing the challenge you identified. Break down your goal into smaller, manageable steps and take consistent action each day. Remember, every small step you take is a victory.

Step 7: Celebrate Your Progress As you take action and make progress, be sure to celebrate your successes along the way. Acknowledging your achievements, no matter how small, reinforces positive behavior and keeps you motivated to continue moving forward.

Remember: Reframing is not about denying the reality of a challenging situation. It's about choosing how you interpret and respond to it. By reframing your thoughts, you empower yourself to take control of your emotions, your decisions, and ultimately, your life.

This exercise is not a one-time fix. It's a practice that requires ongoing effort and commitment. But with time and perseverance, you'll develop a more resilient mindset, overcome your fears, and create a life that is truly regret-free.

Day 18: Mindfulness Meditation/Gratitude Journal

Ever feel like your mind is a runaway train, constantly jumping from one thought to the next? Worrying about the future, replaying the past, never quite present in the here and now? You're not alone. In our fast-paced, hyper-connected world, it's easy to get swept away by the relentless currents of our thoughts and emotions.

But what if there was a way to get off the train, even for a few moments, and find a sense of calm and clarity amidst the chaos? What if you could tap into an inner reservoir of peace and gratitude, no matter what life throws your way?

That's where mindfulness meditation and gratitude journaling come in. These two powerful practices, when combined, offer a dynamic duo for cultivating inner peace, reducing stress, and fostering a more positive outlook on life.

Think of mindfulness as a mental reset button. It's the practice of paying attention to the present moment without judgment. It's about noticing your thoughts and feelings

without getting caught up in them. Like a muscle, the more you practice
mindfulness, the stronger your ability to stay present and grounded becomes.

Gratitude journaling, on the other hand, is like a spotlight that illuminates the good in your life. It's the practice of regularly acknowledging and appreciating the things you're thankful for, big and small. Research has shown that gratitude can significantly boost happiness, reduce stress, and improve overall well-being.

Together, mindfulness and gratitude create a powerful synergy. Mindfulness helps us become aware of our thoughts and emotions, while gratitude allows us to focus on the positive aspects of our lives. By combining these practices, we can train our minds to be more present, more appreciative, and more resilient in the face of life's challenges.

Today, we're going to deepen our mindfulness practice and explore the transformative power of gratitude journaling. We'll delve into more advanced mindfulness techniques that can take your practice to the next level, and we'll discover how gratitude can be woven into every aspect of your life, not just your journal.

By the end of this chapter, you'll have a greater understanding of how mindfulness and gratitude can work together to create a more peaceful, joyful, and fulfilling life. You'll have new tools for managing stress, cultivating self-awareness, and finding moments of calm amidst the chaos.

So, are you ready to step off the runaway train of your thoughts and find your center? Let's dive in and discover the transformative power of mindfulness and gratitude.

DEEPENING MINDFULNESS PRACTICE

By now, you've dipped your toes into the waters of mindfulness. You've likely experienced the calming effects of basic breathing exercises and focused attention. But mindfulness is like a vast ocean, with depths yet to be explored. It's time to dive deeper and discover more advanced techniques that can transform your relationship with yourself, others, and the world around you.

THE BODY SCAN MEDITATION: A JOURNEY WITHIN

Imagine lying down, closing your eyes, and embarking on a journey through your own body. This is the essence of the body scan meditation. It involves systematically bringing awareness to different parts of your body, noticing any sensations, emotions, or thoughts that arise without judgment.

Starting with your toes, you'll gradually move your attention up through your feet, legs, torso, arms, and head, like a gentle wave washing over your entire being. This practice not only cultivates a deeper connection with your physical self but also helps you become more attuned to subtle signals of stress, tension, or discomfort. By learning to simply observe these sensations without reacting, you can develop a greater sense of calm and equanimity.

MINDFUL WALKING: GROUNDING YOURSELF IN THE PRESENT MOMENT

Walking is often something we do on autopilot, our minds busy with thoughts and worries. Mindful walking invites you to slow down, engage your senses, and truly experience the act of walking.

As you walk, focus your attention on the physical sensations of each step – the contact of your feet with the ground, the movement of your legs, the gentle sway of your arms. Notice the sights, sounds, and smells around you. If your mind starts to wander (which it inevitably will), gently bring it back to the sensations of walking.

This practice can help you feel more grounded and centered, reduce stress, and even spark creative insights. It's a simple yet powerful way to incorporate mindfulness into your daily routine, whether it's a walk in nature, a stroll around the block, or even your daily commute.

LOVINGKINDNESS MEDITATION: CULTIVATING COMPASSION

Lovingkindness meditation, also known as Metta meditation, is a practice of cultivating compassion and kindness towards ourselves and others. It involves silently repeating phrases that express well-wishes for happiness, health, and well-being.

You might start by directing these phrases towards yourself, then gradually expand your circle of compassion to include loved ones, acquaintances, strangers, and even those you find difficult. This practice can help dissolve feelings of anger, resentment, and judgment, replacing them with kindness, empathy, and connection.

Research suggests that loving-kindness meditation can reduce stress, increase positive emotions, and even improve our physical health. It's a powerful way to nurture our innate capacity for compassion and create a more harmonious relationship with ourselves and others.

WHY THESE TECHNIQUES MATTER

These advanced mindfulness practices offer a deeper dive into the transformative power of mindfulness. They help you cultivate:

- **Self-awareness:** By paying attention to your body, thoughts, and emotions, you gain a greater understanding of your inner landscape.
- **Emotional regulation:** You learn to observe your emotions without getting overwhelmed by them, developing greater emotional resilience.
- **Compassion:** You cultivate kindness and understanding towards yourself and others, leading to more fulfilling relationships.
- **Inner peace:** By focusing on the present moment, you find a sense of calm and stillness amidst the busyness of life.
- **Clarity:** You gain mental clarity and focus, enabling you to make better decisions and live more intentionally.

INTEGRATING INTO YOUR LIFE

Experiment with these techniques and see which ones resonate with you. You might find that one practice is particularly helpful
for reducing stress, while another is more effective for cultivating compassion.

Incorporate these practices into your daily routine, even if it's just for a few minutes at a time. Remember, consistency is key. The more you practice, the deeper your experience of mindfulness will become.

And most importantly, be patient and kind to yourself. Mindfulness is a journey, not a destination. There will be days when your mind wanders, when you feel restless or distracted. That's okay. Simply acknowledge it and gently guide your attention back to the present moment.

As you continue to deepen your mindfulness practice, you'll discover a greater sense of inner peace, clarity, and connection to yourself and the world around you.

GRATITUDE AS A WAY OF LIFE

Gratitude isn't just a feeling; it's a way of life. It's not confined to the pages of your journal or a fleeting emotion you feel during a specific exercise. It's a mindset, a habit, a conscious choice to see the good in every day, even amidst the challenges.

Now that you've established a gratitude journaling practice, let's explore how you can weave this powerful emotion into the fabric of your daily life. Because gratitude isn't just about *feeling* thankful; it's about *expressing* and *living* that thankfulness in every moment.

EXPRESSING GRATITUDE TO OTHERS

One of the most powerful ways to cultivate gratitude is by expressing it to others. We often forget to tell the people in our lives how much they mean to us, how much we appreciate their support, or how much we value their presence.

So, let's start making a conscious effort to say "thank you." Thank your partner for making you coffee, your colleague for their help on a project, or a stranger for holding the door open for you. These small acts of appreciation may seem insignificant, but they can have a ripple effect, spreading positivity and kindness throughout your day.

Take it a step further and write a heartfelt letter to someone who has made a difference in your life. Share specific examples of how their actions, words, or simply their presence have impacted you. Not only will this express your gratitude, but it will also strengthen your relationship with that person.

SAVORING POSITIVE EXPERIENCES

Life is a collection of moments, both big and small. It's easy to get caught up in the hustle and bustle of everyday life and miss the beauty that surrounds us.

Practicing gratitude invites us to slow down and savor those positive experiences. Notice the warmth of the sun on your skin, the taste of your morning coffee, the sound of your child's laughter. These seemingly mundane moments are filled with joy and wonder when we take the time to appreciate them.

When something good happens, don't just let it pass by. Pause for a moment and truly soak it in. Feel the happiness, the

excitement, the sense of accomplishment. This practice not only amplifies the positive emotions in the moment but also creates lasting memories that you can draw upon in the future.

APPRECIATING THE SMALL JOYS

In our pursuit of big goals and dreams, it's easy to overlook the small joys that make up our daily lives. But it's often those little things that bring us the most happiness.

The smell of freshly baked bread, a vibrant sunset, a cozy conversation with a friend – these seemingly insignificant moments can have a profound impact on our mood and well-being.

Take a few minutes each day to intentionally seek out and appreciate the small joys in your life. It could be as simple as noticing the blooming flowers on your morning walk, enjoying a cup of tea, or listening to your favorite song. By focusing on these small pleasures, you'll cultivate a greater sense of contentment and joy in your everyday life.

GRATITUDE AS A LIFESTYLE

As you continue to weave gratitude into your daily life, you'll find that it becomes less of a conscious effort and more of a natural way of being. You'll start to see the world through a different lens, one that focuses on the good, the positive, and the abundance that surrounds you.

Gratitude is not about ignoring the challenges or denying the difficult emotions that arise. It's about acknowledging them while also choosing to focus on the blessings in your life. It's about recognizing that even in the midst of adversity, there is always something to be thankful for.

Living with gratitude is a gift you give yourself. It's a powerful tool for cultivating happiness, resilience, and a deeper connection to yourself and the world around you. So let's embrace gratitude as a way of life, not just for the next 30 days, but for every day that follows.

EXERCISE: GRATITUDE WALK

Ready to take your gratitude practice to the next level? Let's step outside and embark on a gratitude walk. This isn't about speed or distance; it's about slowing down, tuning in, and opening your heart to the abundance that surrounds you.

PREPARING FOR YOUR WALK

Before you head out, take a few moments to center yourself. Close your eyes, take a few deep breaths, and set an intention for your walk. You might say to yourself, "I am open to receiving the gifts of this moment" or "I am grateful for the opportunity to experience this walk."

Now, lace up your shoes, grab a notebook and pen (optional), and head outside.

Step 1: Engage Your Senses As you begin your walk, slow down your pace and consciously engage your senses. Notice the sights, sounds, smells, and sensations around you.

- **Sight:** Pay attention to the colors of the sky, the leaves on the trees, the patterns of the clouds. Admire the architecture of the buildings, the vibrant flowers, or the playful animals you encounter.
- **Sound:** Listen to the birds singing, the wind rustling through the leaves, the laughter of children playing. Notice the hum of traffic, the chatter of people passing by, or the gentle lapping of waves against the shore.
- **Smell:** Inhale the fresh air, the scent of blooming flowers, the aroma of freshly brewed coffee. Be aware of the earthy smell of soil, the salty air near the ocean, or the comforting scent of home.
- **Touch:** Feel the warmth of the sun on your skin, the cool breeze on your face, the softness of the grass beneath your feet. Notice the texture of the sidewalk, the roughness of tree bark, or the smoothness of a pebble.

Step 2: Express Gratitude As you walk, begin to express gratitude for the things you notice. Start with simple phrases:

- "I am grateful for the blue sky."
- "I am thankful for the sound of the birds singing."
- "I appreciate the sweet smell of the flowers."
- "I am grateful for the warmth of the sun on my skin."

Allow yourself to feel the gratitude in your heart as you speak these words. Let it fill you with warmth and appreciation.

As you continue your walk, your expressions of gratitude can become more elaborate:

- "I am so grateful for the opportunity to take this walk and experience the beauty of nature."
- "I am thankful for my healthy body that allows me to move and explore."
- "I appreciate the kindness of strangers who smile and say hello."
- "I am grateful for the challenges in my life that have helped me grow and become stronger."

Step 3: Journal Your Gratitude *(Optional)* If you've brought a notebook, take a few moments to jot down your observations and expressions of gratitude. This will help you to solidify the experience and create a lasting record of your gratitude walk.

Step 4: Reflect and Continue As you continue your walk, allow your mind to wander and reflect on your experiences. Notice any shifts in your mood, energy levels, or overall sense of well-being.

Remember, gratitude is a muscle that needs to be exercised regularly. The more you practice gratitude, the more naturally it will come to you. Make gratitude walks a regular part of your routine, whether it's a daily stroll around the block or a weekly hike in nature.

BEYOND THE WALK

The benefits of gratitude extend far beyond your walk. As you integrate gratitude into your daily life, you'll start to notice a shift in your perspective. You'll become more attuned to the positive aspects of your life, less focused on what's lacking, and more resilient in the face of challenges.

Gratitude is a powerful tool for cultivating happiness, reducing stress, and improving overall well-being. It's a simple yet profound practice that can transform your life from the inside out. So, take the time to savor the simple joys, appreciate the beauty around you, and express gratitude for the many blessings in your life.

Your journey to a more fulfilling and joyful life begins with one grateful step at a time.

Day 19: Small Wins Celebration

Let's be honest for a minute: big goals can feel overwhelming. The thought of running a marathon, starting a business, or writing a book can seem daunting, even impossible at times. It's easy to get caught up in the grand vision and forget to appreciate the small, incremental steps that lead us there.

But here's the secret: those small wins matter. A lot.

Each time you lace up your running shoes and hit the pavement, you're one step closer to that finish line. Every word you write brings you closer to completing that manuscript. Every client you land or sale you make is a building block in your entrepreneurial journey.

These small victories may seem insignificant in the grand scheme of things, but they're actually the fuel that keeps you going. They provide a sense of accomplishment, boost your confidence, and reinforce your commitment to your goals.

Think of it this way: imagine climbing a mountain. The summit may be your ultimate goal, but you don't just magically teleport there. You have to take one step at a time, conquering each incline, each rocky path, each switchback. And with each step, you get a little closer to the top.

The same is true for any goal you set. It's the accumulation of small wins that propels you forward and makes the seemingly impossible become achievable.

So why don't we celebrate these small wins more often? Why do we wait until we've reached the finish line to pat ourselves on the back?

Perhaps it's because we're conditioned to focus on the end result, rather than the journey. We're taught to strive for perfection, to compare ourselves to others, and to downplay our own achievements.

But it's time to change that narrative.

Today, we're going to celebrate your progress. We're going to acknowledge the small wins you've achieved so far, no matter how insignificant they may seem. We're going to shift our focus from what's left to be done to what's already been accomplished.

Because every step forward, no matter how small, is a victory worth celebrating.

RECOGNIZING PROGRESS

Raise your hand if you've ever felt like your goals were light-years away, the journey endless, and your efforts like a drop in the ocean. (I'm raising my hand right along with you!) It's natural to get caught up in the grand vision of where you want to be, but it's equally important, if not more so, to celebrate the milestones you pass along the way.

I'm not talking about throwing confetti for every little

task you check off your to-do list. But I am talking about recognizing and appreciating the small victories that often get overlooked in our pursuit of bigger goals.

Think of it like hiking a mountain. Sure, the summit is the ultimate prize, the panoramic view that makes all the sweat and sore muscles worthwhile. But what about those breathtaking overlooks along the trail? The wildflowers blooming at your feet? The satisfying crunch of leaves under your boots? These are the small wins that make the journey enjoyable, keep you motivated, and give you the confidence to keep climbing.

THE SCIENCE OF SMALL WINS

Celebrating small wins isn't just about feeling good (though that's a definite perk!). There's actual science behind why it's so effective for personal growth and achieving our goals.

1. **Boosting Motivation:** When we acknowledge our progress, our brains release dopamine, a neurotransmitter associated with pleasure and reward. This positive reinforcement creates a sense of accomplishment and motivates us to continue taking steps toward our goals.
2. **Increasing Self-Efficacy:** Each small win reinforces our belief in our own abilities. As we see ourselves making progress, we become more confident in our skills and our capacity for growth. This increased self-efficacy propels us forward, even when faced with challenges.
3. **Reinforcing Positive Behavior:** Celebrating small wins creates a positive feedback loop. By rewarding

ourselves for taking action, we're more likely to repeat those actions in the future. This builds momentum and makes it easier to establish healthy habits that support our goals.
4. **Building Resilience:** Acknowledging our progress helps us see setbacks as temporary bumps in the road rather than major failures. This builds resilience and enables us to bounce back from challenges more quickly.

HOW TO CELEBRATE YOUR SMALL WINS

Celebrating small wins doesn't have to be elaborate or expensive. It's about finding what works for you and making it a regular practice. Here are a few ideas to get you started:

- **Write it down:** Keep a "win journal" to track your progress and reflect on your achievements.
- **Treat yourself:** Enjoy a small reward, like a cup of your favorite coffee, a relaxing bath, or a fun activity.
- **Share your wins:** Tell a friend, family member, or mentor about your accomplishments. Celebrate together!
- **Do a happy dance:** Seriously, let loose and celebrate! Movement can boost your mood and reinforce the positive feelings associated with your success.
- **Take a break:** Sometimes the best way to celebrate is to simply pause and appreciate the moment. Give yourself permission to rest and recharge.

Remember: There's no such thing as a win that's too small to celebrate. Every step forward, no matter how tiny, is a testament to your effort, your resilience, and your commitment to growth.

So, as you continue on your journey to "No More What Ifs," be sure to pause and acknowledge your progress along the way. Celebrate those small wins, savor the feeling of accomplishment, and let it fuel your motivation to keep moving forward. Remember, even the longest journeys are made one step at a time.

THE POWER OF POSITIVE REINFORCEMENT

Let's talk about celebrations. Not the big, blowout kind with confetti and champagne (though those are fun too!), but the everyday kind that happens when you acknowledge and reward yourself for your achievements.

Think about it: When was the last time you truly celebrated a win, no matter how small? Maybe you finished a challenging project at work, cooked a delicious meal, or simply made it to your morning yoga class. Did you take a moment to savor that feeling of accomplishment? Or did you quickly move on to the next task on your to-do list without a second thought?

In our fast-paced, achievement-oriented society, it's easy to downplay our successes. We're often so focused on what we haven't yet accomplished that we forget to acknowledge how far we've come. But celebrating our wins, no matter how small, is a crucial part of living with intention and cultivating a positive mindset.

THE SCIENCE BEHIND POSITIVE REINFORCEMENT

Positive reinforcement is a powerful psychological principle that explains how our behavior is shaped by rewards and consequences. When we receive a reward for a particular action, we're more likely to repeat that action in the future. This creates a positive feedback loop that encourages further progress and reinforces positive behavior.

Think about it like training a dog. When the dog sits on command, you give it a treat. The dog learns that sitting leads to a reward, so it's more likely to sit again in the future. The same principle applies to humans. When we celebrate our wins, we're essentially giving ourselves a "treat." This reinforces the positive behavior that led to the success, making us more likely to repeat it.

CELEBRATING SMALL WINS: A CATALYST FOR GROWTH

Celebrating small wins isn't just about feeling good in the moment; it's about creating a sustainable cycle of growth and progress. When we acknowledge and reward ourselves for our efforts, we boost our motivation, increase our self-efficacy (our belief in our own abilities), and strengthen our resilience in the face of challenges.

Each small win serves as a stepping stone towards our larger goals. By celebrating each step along the way, we build momentum and create a positive spiral of success. The more we acknowledge our progress, the more motivated we become to keep going. And the more motivated we are, the more likely we are to achieve our goals.

CELEBRATING YOUR WAY

Celebrating wins doesn't have to be a big production. It can be as simple as taking a few moments to pat yourself on the back, journaling about your accomplishment, or sharing your success with a friend or loved one.

The key is to find what feels authentic and meaningful to you. Maybe you enjoy treating yourself to a special meal, buying yourself a small gift, or simply taking a break to relax and recharge. Whatever it is, make sure it's something that makes you feel good and reinforces the positive behavior.

Here are a few more ideas for celebrating your wins:

- **Write down your accomplishment:** Keep a "wins journal" where you record your successes, no matter how small.
- **Share your wins with others:** Tell a friend, family member, or colleague about your achievement. Let them celebrate with you!
- **Create a visual reminder:** Hang up a certificate, post a picture of yourself achieving your goal, or create a visual representation of your progress.
- **Do something you enjoy:** Take some time to engage in an activity you love, whether it's reading, listening to music, spending time in nature, or simply relaxing with a cup of tea.
- **Set a new goal:** Use the momentum of your win to set a

new, slightly more challenging goal. This will keep you moving forward and striving for continued growth.

THE BOTTOM LINE

Celebrating your successes, no matter how small, is not about being self-centered or boastful. It's about recognizing your effort, appreciating your progress, and fueling your motivation to keep going. It's about creating a positive feedback loop that reinforces positive behavior and leads to lasting change.

So, the next time you achieve a goal, no matter how small it may seem, take a moment to celebrate. Acknowledge your hard work, savor the feeling of accomplishment, and use that energy to propel you forward on your journey to a more intentional and fulfilling life. Remember, every step you take, no matter how small, is a victory worth celebrating.

EXERCISE: SMALL WINS REFLECTION

Take a deep breath, friend. We've covered a lot of ground in the past few weeks. We've faced our fears head-on, confronted our regrets, and started making intentional choices aligned with our purpose. That's a lot to celebrate!

But hold on a second. Before we dive into the final stretch of this journey, let's take a moment to acknowledge and

appreciate the progress you've already made. It's easy to get caught up in the big picture, focusing only on the ultimate destination. But the truth is, every step of this journey is worth celebrating.

WHY SMALL WINS MATTER

Think back to the beginning of this book. Remember those moments when fear and regret held you back? Remember the self-doubt that whispered in your ear, telling you that you weren't good enough, strong enough, or worthy enough?

You've come a long way since then. You've learned to challenge those negative thoughts, reframe your perspective, and take small but significant steps toward your goals. Each of those steps, no matter how small, is a victory. It's a testament to your courage, resilience, and commitment to creating a better life.

Celebrating small wins is not about vanity or self-indulgence. It's about acknowledging your progress, boosting your confidence, and reinforcing positive behavior. When we take the time to appreciate our achievements, we fuel our motivation and create a positive feedback loop that encourages us to keep moving forward.

YOUR SMALL WINS REFLECTION

Take a few moments now to reflect on the past week. Think about the challenges you've faced, the decisions you've made, and the actions you've taken. What were some of the small wins you achieved?

Maybe you...

- Spoke up in a meeting when you usually stay quiet.
- Tried a new recipe you've been wanting to make.

- Went for a walk instead of scrolling through social media.
- Reached out to a friend you haven't spoken to in a while.
- Completed a task you've been procrastinating on.
- Wore an outfit that made you feel confident.
- Practiced mindfulness for five minutes without getting distracted.
- Said "no" to something that wasn't aligned with your values.
- Forgave yourself for a past mistake.
- Took a step towards your dream career.

No matter how small it may seem, each of these actions is a win. It's a step in the right direction, a sign of progress, and a reason to celebrate.

CELEBRATING YOUR WINS

Now that you've identified your small wins, it's time to celebrate them. How you choose to celebrate is entirely up to you. There's no right or wrong way to do it. The most important thing is to choose a celebration that feels meaningful and authentic to you.

Here are a few ideas to get you started:

- **Write it down:** Take a few minutes to journal about your wins. Describe what you accomplished, how it made you feel, and what you learned from the experience.

- **Treat yourself:** Indulge in something you enjoy, whether it's a cup of coffee, a relaxing bath, or a new book.
- **Share your wins:** Tell a friend, family member, or mentor about your achievements. Sharing your successes with others can amplify the positive feelings and create a sense of accountability.
- **Do a happy dance:** Put on your favorite music and let loose! Express your joy and celebrate your accomplishments through movement.
- **Create a "wins jar":** Write down your wins on slips of paper and put them in a jar. At the end of the month, read through your wins and reflect on your progress.
- **Reward yourself:** Set up a reward system for yourself. For example, after achieving a certain number of small wins, treat yourself to a special outing or experience.
- **Simply acknowledge it:** Take a moment to pause, reflect, and acknowledge your achievement. Say to yourself, "I did it!" and feel the pride and satisfaction that comes with accomplishment.

KEEP THE MOMENTUM GOING

Remember, celebrating your wins is not just about feeling good in the moment. It's about building momentum, reinforcing positive behavior, and creating a habit of recognizing and appreciating your progress.

As you continue on your journey, make celebrating small wins a regular practice. By acknowledging your achievements and giving yourself credit for the effort you put in, you'll cultivate a sense of self-efficacy and confidence that will propel you towards even greater success.

Day 20: Vision Board Completion

Remember that dream you've been holding onto? That vision of your future that makes your heart race a little faster? Today, we're turning those dreams into tangible aspirations with the final touches on your vision board.

Over the past few days, you've gathered images, words, and quotes that reflect your deepest desires, values, and goals. You've explored what truly lights you up and identified the steps needed to create a life that aligns with your purpose. Now, it's time to bring those aspirations to life by completing your vision board.

Your vision board is more than just a collage of pretty pictures; it's a powerful tool for manifestation. It's a visual representation of your goals and dreams, a constant reminder of what you're working towards, and a source of inspiration to keep you motivated and focused.

By creating a vision board, you're essentially telling your subconscious mind, "This is what I want. This is where I'm going." And your subconscious, in turn, will start working tirelessly to help you achieve those goals. It's like planting seeds

in fertile soil; with the right care and attention, they will eventually bloom into reality.

THE FINAL TOUCHES

Today, take some time to review your vision board and make any final adjustments. Are there any missing pieces? Any areas that need more clarity or focus? Add any additional images, words, or quotes that resonate with you and reflect your evolving aspirations.

Don't be afraid to get creative and personalize your board. Use colors, textures, and patterns that inspire you. Make it a reflection of your unique personality and style. Remember, this is your vision, so make it yours!

ACTIVATING YOUR VISION

Once your vision board is complete, it's time to activate it. This means more than just hanging it on your wall; it's about infusing it with your energy, intention, and belief.

Find a prominent place in your home or workspace where you'll see your vision board every day. Make it a part of your daily routine to spend a few minutes looking at it, visualizing your goals as if they've already been achieved. Feel the excitement, joy, and gratitude as if you're already living your dream life.

Remember, your vision board is a living document. It can evolve and change as you do. Don't hesitate to update it periodically with new images, goals, or aspirations. The key is to keep it relevant and inspiring so that it continues to serve as a powerful motivator on your journey.

As you engage with your vision board, you'll notice a shift in your mindset. You'll start to see opportunities and possibilities that you may have missed before. You'll find yourself taking actions that align with your goals and attracting the resources and support you need to make your dreams a reality.

So go ahead and unleash the power of your vision board. Let it be your roadmap to a life of purpose, passion, and no regrets.

THE FINAL TOUCHES

By now, your vision board should be well on its way to reflecting the vibrant future you're creating. It's a collage of hopes, dreams, and aspirations, each image and word carefully chosen to represent what truly matters to you. But before we move on to activating this powerful tool, let's add those final touches that will make your vision board sing.

Think of your vision board as a masterpiece in progress. It's time to add those last few brushstrokes that will make it pop with personality and truly reflect your unique essence. Remember, this is *your* vision, so don't be afraid to let your creativity flow!

FILLING IN THE GAPS

Take a good look at your board. Are there any areas that feel a little empty or unbalanced? Perhaps there's a specific goal that hasn't been fully represented, or maybe you want to add a touch of whimsy to lighten the mood. Now's the time to fill those gaps with additional images, words, or quotes that resonate with you.

Don't limit yourself to just pictures. Consider adding words or phrases that capture your aspirations, values, or desired emotions. These could be words like "joy," "abundance," "freedom," or phrases like "living my best life," "following my dreams," or "making a difference."

THE POWER OF QUOTES

Quotes are a fantastic way to add a touch of inspiration and wisdom to your vision board. They can serve as daily reminders of your goals, reinforce positive beliefs, or simply provide a boost of motivation when you need it most.

Search for quotes that resonate with your vision. You can find them online, in books, or even in your own journal. Look for quotes that speak to your heart, challenge you to grow, or simply make you smile.

A TOUCH OF PERSONALIZATION

Your vision board should be a reflection of you. Add elements that showcase your personality, interests, and unique style. This could include photos of loved ones, meaningful objects, or even a splash of your favorite color.

Consider using different textures or materials to make your board more visually appealing. You can add ribbons, fabric scraps, stickers, glitter, or anything else that sparks your creativity. The goal is to create a board that you'll enjoy looking at every day and that feels truly yours.

MAKING IT PRETTY

Don't underestimate the power of aesthetics. A visually appealing vision board can uplift your spirits, spark your imagination, and make you feel more connected to your dreams. Take the time to arrange your images and words in a way that is pleasing to the eye.

Experiment with different layouts and arrangements until you find one that feels just right. You can group similar items together, create a theme, or simply let your intuition guide you.

Tips for Creating a Visually Appealing Vision Board:

- **Use high-quality images:** Choose images that are clear, vibrant, and visually striking.
- **Balance colors and textures:** Create a visually interesting composition by combining different colors and textures.
- **Leave some white space:** Avoid overcrowding your board. Leave some blank space to give your eyes a rest and allow each image to shine.
- **Get creative:** Don't be afraid to experiment with different materials, layouts, and styles.
- **Make it personal:** Add elements that reflect your unique personality and interests.

Remember, your vision board is a living document. It can evolve and change as your goals and dreams shift. Don't be afraid to add new elements or remove old ones as needed. The most important thing is that your vision board inspires and motivates you to take action towards your dreams.

ACTIVATING YOUR VISION

Your vision board isn't just a pretty collage; it's a powerful tool designed to ignite your motivation, focus your energy, and manifest your dreams into reality. Think of it as a daily dose of inspiration, a visual reminder of the life you're creating, and a roadmap to your goals.

Now that your vision board is complete, it's time to breathe life into it. But how do you actually *use* it to make a tangible difference in your life? Here's where the magic happens:

1. **Strategic Placement:** Don't tuck your vision board away in a drawer or closet! Place it somewhere you'll see it every single day. This could be on your bedroom wall, next to your desk, or even as the background on your phone or computer. The key is to make it a constant presence in your life.
2. **Daily Ritual:** Set aside a few minutes each day to connect with your vision board. This could be first thing in the morning, during your lunch break, or before bed. There's no right or wrong time, as long as it's consistent.
3. **Engage Your Senses:** As you look at your vision board, take a deep breath and allow yourself to fully *feel* the

emotions associated with your dreams. See yourself achieving those goals, experiencing those successes, and living that life you've envisioned.

4. **Visualize with Detail:** Don't just glance at your board; dive deep into the details. Imagine the sights, sounds, smells, and tastes associated with your goals. The more vivid your visualization, the more powerful it becomes.

5. **Affirm Your Desires:** As you visualize, repeat affirmations that reinforce your commitment to your goals. For example, if your board features a picture of a dream home, you might say, "I am attracting my perfect home into my life."

6. **Feel the Excitement:** Allow yourself to feel the excitement, joy, and gratitude that come with achieving your dreams. This positive energy will fuel your actions and propel you forward.

7. **Take Inspired Action:** Your vision board is not a passive tool; it's a call to action. After visualizing your goals, ask yourself, "What can I do today to move closer to my dreams?" Then, take one small step, no matter how small, in the direction of your vision.

8. **Update and Evolve:** Your vision board is not set in stone. As you grow and evolve, so too will your dreams and aspirations. Feel free to update your board regularly, adding new images or removing ones that no longer resonate with you.

THE SCIENCE BEHIND VISION BOARDS

You might be wondering, "Does this visualization stuff really
work?" The answer is a resounding yes! There's a growing body of research that supports the power of visualization in achieving our goals.

When we visualize our desired outcomes, our brains create neural pathways as if we were actually experiencing those outcomes. This primes our minds for success and increases our motivation to take action. It's like planting a seed in our subconscious mind that begins to grow and flourish.

Furthermore, vision boards tap into the power of the Reticular Activating System (RAS), a part of our brain that filters information and brings to our attention things that are important to us. When we create a vision board and focus on our goals, we activate the RAS, making us more likely to notice opportunities and resources that can help us achieve those goals.

ADDITIONAL TIPS FOR ACTIVATING YOUR VISION

Here are a few additional tips to make the most of your vision board:

- **Share Your Vision:** Talk about your goals and dreams with supportive friends, family, or a mentor. Sharing your vision can create a sense of accountability and encourage you to stay on track.

- **Create a Vision Board Buddy:** Partner up with a friend and share your vision boards with each other. Encourage and support each other on your journeys.
- **Make it Fun:** Don't take your vision board too seriously. Let it be a source of joy and inspiration. Add elements that make you smile or laugh.

Remember, your vision board is a living, breathing representation of your dreams. It's a tool that can help you create a life of purpose, passion, and fulfillment. So embrace it, use it, and watch as your dreams become your reality.

EXERCISE: VISION BOARD RITUAL

Your vision board is more than just a collage of pretty pictures. It's a powerful tool for manifesting your dreams and goals. But like any tool, its effectiveness depends on how you use it. That's why I want to introduce you to the concept of a vision board ritual.

A vision board ritual is a simple yet powerful way to connect with your vision and infuse it with energy and intention. It's a sacred practice that helps you visualize your dreams as if they are already happening, making them feel more tangible and achievable. By creating a ritual around your vision board, you transform it from a static object into a dynamic catalyst for change.

Why create a ritual? Rituals have been used for centuries across cultures to mark important transitions, connect with the sacred, and create a sense of focus and intention. They have a way of anchoring us in the present moment and activating our inner power. By creating a ritual around your vision board, you tap into this ancient wisdom and harness its power to manifest your dreams.

CRAFTING YOUR VISION BOARD RITUAL

Your ritual can be as simple or elaborate as you like. There's no right or wrong way to do it. The most important thing is that it feels meaningful and inspiring to you. Here are a few ideas to get you started:

- **Create a Sacred Space:** Choose a quiet, peaceful place where you won't be interrupted. You might want to decorate your space with candles, crystals, or other objects that hold significance for you.
- **Set the Mood:** Dim the lights, put on some calming music, or diffuse essential oils that promote relaxation and focus.
- **Light a Candle:** Lighting a candle can symbolize your intention to illuminate your path and bring your dreams to life.
- **Take a Few Deep Breaths:** Center yourself by taking a few deep breaths. Inhale slowly and deeply, feeling your belly expand. Exhale slowly, releasing any tension or worry.
- **Express Gratitude:** Take a moment to express gratitude for the present moment and all the blessings in your life. This helps to shift your focus from lack to abundance.
- **Recite Affirmations:** Choose affirmations that align

with your goals and dreams. Say them out loud with conviction, feeling the truth of the words in your body.
- **Connect with Your Vision Board:** Gaze at your vision board, allowing yourself to feel the emotions associated with each image or word. Imagine yourself living the life you desire, as if it's already happening.
- **Close with Gratitude:** Thank the universe, your higher power, or simply yourself for the opportunity to create this powerful vision.

MAKE IT YOUR OWN

Remember, this is just a starting point. Feel free to personalize your ritual in any way that feels authentic to you. You might want to incorporate movement, music, prayer, or any other practice that helps you connect with your inner wisdom and creativity.

Here are a few additional tips:

- **Choose a Time and Frequency:** Decide how often you want to perform your ritual. You might want to do it daily, weekly, or whenever you feel the need for a boost of inspiration.
- **Keep a Journal:** Keep a journal to record your experiences with the ritual. Write down any insights, feelings, or synchronicities that arise.
- **Be Open to Inspiration:** Pay attention to any messages or signs that come your way during or after your ritual. These could be subtle hints from the universe guiding you towards your goals.

THE POWER OF RITUAL

By creating a vision board ritual, you're not just setting intentions; you're creating a powerful energetic container for your dreams to manifest. You're aligning your thoughts, feelings, and actions with your vision, making it more likely that you'll attract the opportunities and resources you need to achieve your goals.

Remember, the most important thing is to approach your ritual with an open heart and a willingness to believe in the power of your dreams. As you consistently engage with your vision board through this sacred practice, you'll start to see subtle shifts in your mindset, your energy, and the opportunities that come your way.

So go ahead and create your own unique vision board ritual. Let it be a time for you to connect with your deepest desires, ignite your passions, and step into the life you were meant to live.

Part 3: Living a Regret-Free Life (Days 21-30)

Day 21: Integrate Daily Practices

Congratulations! You've reached a significant milestone in your journey to living a regret-free life. Over the past twenty days, you've confronted your fears, explored your purpose, and cultivated empowering habits. Now, it's time to solidify these practices and make them an integral part of your daily life.

Remember that morning jog you used to dread? Or the healthy eating plan you abandoned after a few weeks? The same principle applies to personal growth. Without consistent effort, the initial excitement and motivation can fade, and old habits can creep back in. But fear not! By intentionally integrating the practices you've learned into your routine, you can ensure lasting transformation.

Think of it like this: You've been training for a marathon, and now it's race day. You wouldn't suddenly switch back to your old sedentary lifestyle, right? Similarly, the tools and strategies you've acquired during this 30-day challenge are your training for a life of purpose, passion, and no regrets. It's time to put that training into action.

CREATING YOUR PERSONAL "NO MORE WHAT IFS" ROUTINE

There's no one-size-fits-all approach to integrating these practices. What works for one person might not work for another. The key is to experiment, find what resonates with you, and create a routine that feels sustainable and enjoyable.

Here are some tips to get you started:

- **Schedule it in:** Just like you schedule meetings or appointments, block off time in your calendar for your daily practices. Whether it's 15 minutes for journaling, 10 minutes for meditation, or a few minutes for power poses, make it a non-negotiable part of your day.
- **Start small:** Don't overwhelm yourself by trying to do everything at once. Begin with one or two practices that resonate most with you, and gradually add others as you feel comfortable.
- **Stack habits:** Pair new habits with existing ones to make them easier to remember. For example, you could practice affirmations while brushing your teeth or listen to a motivational podcast during your commute.
- **Find a buddy:** Having a friend or family member join you on your journey can provide accountability and support. Consider sharing your goals and progress with someone who will cheer you on.
- **Be flexible:** Life happens. There will be days when you miss a meditation session or forget to write in your gratitude journal. Don't beat yourself up. Just pick up where you left off and keep moving forward.

- **Celebrate your wins:** Acknowledge and celebrate your progress, no matter how small. Each day that you show up for yourself is a victory.

Remember, this is not about adding more tasks to your already busy schedule. It's about creating a life that is aligned with your values, passions, and purpose. It's about making choices that empower you to live with intention, confidence, and no regrets.

So, are you ready to make "No More What Ifs" your new normal? Let's dive into the next chapter and start integrating these powerful practices into your daily life!

CREATING A ROUTINE

Remember when you were a kid, and your parents insisted on a bedtime routine? Maybe you resisted, but deep down, you knew that brushing your teeth, reading a story, and snuggling into bed helped you feel safe and secure. As adults, we often dismiss routines as boring or restrictive. But the truth is, routines can be incredibly empowering, especially when they're designed to support our well-being and goals.

Think of a routine as a loving embrace you give yourself each day. It's a series of small, intentional actions that nourish your mind, body, and spirit. By incorporating the practices you've learned so far—affirmations, gratitude, mindfulness, and power poses—into a daily routine, you're essentially creating a personalized toolkit for success and happiness.

THE IMPORTANCE OF CONSISTENCY

Let's be honest: change isn't easy. It takes time, effort, and a healthy dose of perseverance. That's where consistency comes in. When you commit to practicing something regularly, you create a ripple effect that gradually transforms your life.

Think of it like this: each time you practice gratitude, you're strengthening your "gratitude muscle." Each time you engage in mindfulness, you're training your brain to focus and be present. And each time you strike a power pose, you're boosting your confidence and reducing stress.

Consistency is key because it helps you build momentum. Just like a snowball rolling down a hill, your small, consistent actions will gather strength and power over time, leading to significant and lasting changes.

BUILDING A ROUTINE THAT WORKS FOR YOU

The beauty of a routine is that it's entirely customizable. There's no one-size-fits-all approach. The key is to create a routine that fits your lifestyle, preferences, and goals.

Here are some tips for building a routine that works for you:

1. **Start Small:** Don't try to overhaul your entire life overnight. Start by incorporating one or two new practices into your existing routine.
2. **Choose the Right Time:** Think about when you're most likely to be successful with your new habits. Are

you a morning person or a night owl? Do you have more free time on weekends or weekdays?
3. **Be Flexible:** Life happens. There will be days when you can't stick to your routine perfectly. That's okay! Don't beat yourself up. Just pick up where you left off the next day.
4. **Track Your Progress:** Keep a journal or use an app to track your daily practices. This will help you stay accountable and see how far you've come.
5. **Celebrate Your Wins:** Acknowledge your efforts and celebrate your successes, no matter how small. This will help you stay motivated and on track.

YOUR DAILY DOSE OF AWESOME: A SAMPLE ROUTINE

To get you started, here's a sample routine that incorporates the practices you've learned:

- Morning:
    - Wake up and spend 5 minutes doing power poses.
    - Read or listen to your affirmations.
    - Write in your gratitude journal (3 things you're grateful for).
    - Practice mindfulness meditation for 10-15 minutes.
- Throughout the Day:
    - Take short mindfulness breaks to reconnect with the present moment.

- Repeat your affirmations whenever you feel self-doubt creeping in.
- Practice gratitude in your interactions with others.
- If you're feeling stressed or overwhelmed, strike a power pose for a quick confidence boost.
- Evening:
  - Reflect on your day and identify three things that went well.
  - Write in your gratitude journal again (3 things you're grateful for).
  - Do a relaxing activity, such as reading, taking a bath, or listening to calming music.

Remember, this is just a sample routine. Feel free to adjust it to fit your own needs and preferences. The most important thing is to find what works for you and stick with it.

By creating a daily routine that incorporates these powerful practices, you're setting yourself up for success in all areas of your life. You'll build resilience, increase confidence, reduce stress, and cultivate a deeper sense of purpose and fulfillment. So, what are you waiting for? Start creating your daily dose of awesome today!

THE POWER OF RITUALS

Let's talk rituals. Not the elaborate, time-consuming kind that involve chanting or sacrificing chickens (unless that's your thing, of course!). I'm talking about simple, meaningful practices that can transform your everyday routine into a sacred experience.

Think of rituals as intentional acts that anchor you in the present moment, connect you to your values, and infuse your life with a deeper sense of purpose. They're not about adding more to your to-do list, but rather about infusing existing activities with intention and significance.

WHY RITUALS MATTER

Rituals have been a part of human culture for centuries. From religious ceremonies to cultural traditions, rituals have served

as a way to mark important life transitions, connect with the divine, and create a sense of community and belonging.

But rituals aren't just for special occasions. They can be woven into the fabric of our daily lives, adding a layer of richness and meaning to even the most mundane tasks. Here's why rituals are so powerful:

- They create a sense of grounding and stability. In a world that often feels chaotic and unpredictable, rituals offer a sense of predictability and routine. They create a framework for our day and help us feel more grounded and centered.
- They connect us to our values and purpose. By intentionally choosing rituals that align with our values and goals, we reinforce our commitment to living a purposeful life. Every time we perform a ritual, we're reminded of what truly matters to us.

- They enhance our focus and concentration. Rituals can help us clear our minds, quiet the mental chatter, and focus our attention on the task at hand. This can be particularly beneficial for activities that require deep concentration, such as work or creative projects.
- They reduce stress and anxiety. By creating a sense of order and predictability, rituals can help us feel more in control and less overwhelmed by life's challenges. They can also provide a much-needed pause from the hustle and bustle of daily life.
- They cultivate gratitude and mindfulness. Many rituals involve elements of gratitude and mindfulness, such as taking a few moments to appreciate the simple things in life or focusing on our breath. These practices can have a profound impact on our overall well-being.

RITUALS FOR A PURPOSEFUL LIFE

Now that we understand the power of rituals, let's explore a few simple practices that you can incorporate into your daily life to start and end your day with intention:

- **Morning Affirmations:** Start your day by reciting positive affirmations that align with your purpose and goals. This could be as simple as saying, "I am capable," "I am worthy," or "I am living my purpose."
- **Vision Board Ritual:** Take a few minutes each morning to gaze at your vision board and visualize your dreams coming true. This will help you stay connected to your goals and fuel your motivation throughout the day.

- **Gratitude Practice Before Bed:** Before you drift off to sleep, take a few moments to reflect on the day and express gratitude for the good things that happened. This could involve writing in a gratitude journal, listing three things you're thankful for, or simply saying a silent prayer of thanks.

These are just a few examples of rituals that you can incorporate into your daily life. The most important thing is to choose practices that resonate with you and that you can commit to doing consistently.

CREATING YOUR OWN RITUALS

As you experiment with different rituals, remember that there are no right or wrong answers. The most effective rituals are the ones that feel authentic and meaningful to you. Here are a few tips for creating your own rituals:

- **Start small:** Don't feel like you need to overhaul your entire routine overnight. Start by incorporating one or two small rituals into your day and gradually add more as you feel comfortable.
- **Choose rituals that align with your values and goals:** Your rituals should serve as a reminder of what's important to you and what you're working towards.
- **Make them enjoyable:** Your rituals should be something you look forward to, not another chore on your to-do list. Choose activities that bring you joy and peace.

- **Be consistent:** The power of rituals lies in their repetition. Make a commitment to practicing your rituals regularly, even when you don't feel like it.
- **Be open to change:** Your rituals may evolve and change over time as you grow and evolve. That's okay! Be flexible and allow your rituals to adapt to your changing needs and preferences.

Remember, the goal of creating rituals is not to add more stress or pressure to your life. It's about finding simple, meaningful ways to connect with your purpose, cultivate gratitude, and live each day with intention. By incorporating rituals into your daily routine, you'll be surprised at how much more grounded,

focused, and fulfilled you will feel. So, start experimenting today and discover the transformative power of rituals in your own life.

EXERCISE: DESIGN YOUR DAILY RITUALS

Alright, my friend, let's get practical. It's time to take all the amazing tools you've gathered over the past 29 days and weave them into the fabric of your everyday life. This is where the rubber meets the road, where intention transforms from a concept into a lived experience.

Remember, this isn't about following a rigid schedule or adhering to someone else's idea of a "perfect" routine. It's about crafting a rhythm that resonates with your unique needs, preferences, and lifestyle. Think of it as designing a personalized roadmap for intentional living, a roadmap that will guide you towards your goals, nurture your well-being, and infuse your days with purpose and meaning.

WHERE TO BEGIN?

1. **Reflect on Your Values:** Start by revisiting your core values. What matters most to you? What principles do you want to guide your life? Your daily rituals should be a reflection of these values, helping you embody them in every action you take.
2. **Identify Your Non-Negotiables:** What are the practices that have resonated most with you during this 30-day journey? Is it your morning affirmations, your gratitude practice, or your mindfulness meditation? Choose a few non-negotiable rituals that you commit to practicing every day.
3. **Consider Your Schedule and Lifestyle:** Be realistic about your daily schedule and commitments. Are you a morning person or a night owl? Do you have children, a demanding job, or other responsibilities? Tailor your rituals to fit your lifestyle, not the other way around.
4. **Experiment and Adapt:** Don't be afraid to experiment with different rituals and timings. Try adding a new practice to your morning routine or creating a calming ritual before bed. See what feels good, what supports your well-being, and what helps you stay connected to your purpose.

BUILDING YOUR RITUALS

Here are some ideas to get you started, but feel free to customize them to fit your own unique needs:

- Morning Rituals:
    - Start with a few minutes of quiet reflection or meditation.
    - Read or listen to something inspiring.
    - Write in your gratitude journal.
    - Repeat your affirmations.
    - Set your intention for the day.
- Midday Rituals:
    - Take a mindful break from work or chores.
    - Go for a walk in nature.
    - Listen to uplifting music.
    - Connect with a loved one.
- Evening Rituals:
    - Disconnect from technology and wind down.
    - Reflect on your day and practice gratitude.
    - Read or listen to something relaxing.
    - Prepare for a restful sleep.

The Key is Consistency The power of rituals lies in their consistency. By repeating them regularly, they become ingrained habits that support your overall well-being and help you live more intentionally. Remember, it takes time and effort to establish new habits, so be patient with yourself and celebrate each small victory.

Don't be afraid to adjust your rituals as needed. Life is

dynamic, and your needs and priorities may change over time. The key is to remain flexible and adaptable, while still holding onto the core practices that serve you best.

YOUR TURN

Now it's your turn to create your personalized daily rituals. Grab a notebook and pen and start brainstorming. What practices resonate the most with you? How can you integrate them into your daily life in a way that feels sustainable and enjoyable?

Remember, there's no right or wrong way to do this. Trust your intuition, experiment with different approaches, and have fun with it. Your daily rituals should be a source of joy and nourishment, not a burden or a chore.

As you design your rituals, remember that you're not just creating a routine; you're crafting a life. You're building a foundation for intentional living, a life filled with purpose, passion, and joy. So go forth and create a rhythm that supports your dreams and empowers you to live your best life!

Day 22: Embrace Imperfection

Let's be real for a moment: Nobody's perfect. Not you, not me, not even the most seemingly put-together people you see on social media. We all have flaws, make mistakes, and experience setbacks. That's simply part of being human.

Yet, many of us get trapped in the pursuit of perfection. We strive for flawless appearances, impeccable performance, and unwavering success. But this relentless pursuit is not only exhausting, it's also counterproductive.

THE PERFECTIONISM TRAP

Perfectionism is a sneaky little beast. It masquerades as a noble pursuit of excellence, but in reality, it's a fear-driven trap. We worry that if we're not perfect, we won't be loved, accepted, or valued. We fear judgment, criticism, and failure.

This fear of imperfection can lead to procrastination, anxiety, and a crippling self-doubt. We may avoid taking risks, starting new projects, or pursuing our dreams because we're afraid we won't be able to do them perfectly. We may constantly compare ourselves to others, feeling inadequate and never good enough.

The truth is, perfectionism is an illusion. It's an unattainable standard that sets us up for disappointment and frustration. It robs us of the joy of the journey and prevents us from truly embracing our unique selves.

THE BEAUTY OF IMPERFECTION

What if, instead of striving for perfection, we embraced our imperfections? What if we celebrated our flaws as unique qualities that make us who we are? What if we saw mistakes as opportunities for growth and learning, rather than sources of shame?

Embracing imperfection doesn't mean giving up on our goals or settling for mediocrity. It means recognizing that we are human, and as humans, we are inherently imperfect. It means accepting ourselves with all our quirks, idiosyncrasies, and vulnerabilities.

When we let go of the need to be perfect, we open ourselves up to a world of possibilities. We free ourselves from the fear of failure and the pressure to please others. We give ourselves permission to be authentic, to take risks, and to live a life that is true to who we are.

YOUR IMPERFECTLY PERFECT SELF

Today, I invite you to embrace your imperfect, perfectly human self. Celebrate your quirks, your flaws, and your unique way of being in the world. Remember that mistakes are simply stepping stones on the path to growth, and that setbacks are not failures, but opportunities to learn and try again.

By embracing your imperfections, you will not only find greater peace and self-acceptance, but you will also unlock your true potential. You will discover a new level of confidence, creativity, and resilience. You will become a more compassionate and understanding friend, partner, and human being.

So let go of the pursuit of perfection and embrace the beautiful mess that is you. It's in your imperfection that you will find your true strength, your authentic voice, and your most fulfilling life.

THE MYTH OF PERFECTION

Let's be real for a moment: Perfection doesn't exist.

It's a mirage, a fantasy we chase but never truly catch. We've been conditioned to believe that we need to be flawless to be worthy of love, success, or happiness. But here's the secret: that's a lie.

The myth of perfection is a heavy burden to bear. It's like trying to scale a mountain that keeps growing taller with every step you take. It's exhausting, demoralizing, and ultimately, impossible.

Perfectionism isn't about striving for excellence; it's about striving for the unattainable. It's a relentless pursuit of an idealized image that doesn't exist in reality. And when we inevitably fall short of this impossible standard, we beat ourselves up, feel inadequate, and question our worth.

THE DANGERS OF PERFECTIONISM

Perfectionism isn't just a harmless quirk; it can have serious consequences for our mental, emotional, and physical well-being. It's a breeding ground for anxiety, depression, and burnout.

Here's how the myth of perfection can sabotage your happiness:

1. **Procrastination:** Perfectionists often put off starting or finishing tasks because they're afraid of not doing them perfectly. They get caught in a cycle of overthinking, planning, and revising, never feeling quite ready to take action.

2. **Anxiety and Stress:** The pressure to be perfect creates a constant state of anxiety and stress. Perfectionists worry about making mistakes, being judged, or not living up to their own (or others') expectations.

3. **Fear of Failure:** Perfectionists see failure as a personal reflection of their worth. This fear can be paralyzing, preventing them from taking risks or trying new things.

4. **Low Self-Esteem:** The constant comparison to an unattainable ideal leads to feelings of inadequacy and low self-worth. Perfectionists often believe that they're not good enough, no matter how much they achieve.

5. **Burnout:** The relentless pursuit of perfection can lead

to burnout, a state of emotional, physical, and mental exhaustion.

THE ANTIDOTE: EMBRACING IMPERFECTION

The good news is that there's an antidote to perfectionism: embracing imperfection.

This doesn't mean giving up on your goals or settling for mediocrity. It means recognizing that mistakes are a natural part of life and that our imperfections are what make us unique and beautiful.

Embracing imperfection is about:

- **Accepting Yourself:** Acknowledging your strengths and weaknesses, your flaws and your quirks. It's about recognizing that you are worthy of love and respect, just as you are.
- **Focusing on Progress, Not Perfection:** Shifting your focus from the end result to the process of learning and growth. Celebrate small wins and use mistakes as opportunities to learn and improve.
- **Challenging Your Inner Critic:** Notice when your inner critic starts to berate you, and gently remind yourself that you are doing your best. Replace negative self-talk with positive affirmations.
- **Setting Realistic Expectations:** Let go of the need to be perfect in everything you do. Set realistic goals that challenge you but are also attainable.
- **Practicing Self-Compassion:** Treat yourself with the

same kindness and understanding that you would offer a friend. Be patient with yourself, forgive your mistakes, and celebrate your progress.

Embracing imperfection is a journey, not a destination. It takes time, effort, and a willingness to challenge deeply ingrained beliefs. But the rewards are immense. When you let go of the need to be perfect, you free yourself to live a life that is authentic, joyful, and full of possibilities.

THE BEAUTY OF IMPERFECTION

Let's be real here for a moment – none of us are perfect. Not even close. We all have flaws, quirks, and those little (or sometimes not-so-little) imperfections that make us, well, human. And that's okay. In fact, it's more than okay – it's beautiful.

I know, I know, we're constantly bombarded with messages telling us to strive for perfection. Social media feeds filled with flawlessly curated lives, magazines showcasing airbrushed models, and the relentless pressure to be the best version of ourselves can leave us feeling inadequate and insecure. But here's the secret: perfection is an illusion. It doesn't exist.

Chasing after an unattainable ideal is not only exhausting, but it's also counterproductive. When we focus on our perceived flaws, we miss out on the beauty and richness of our unique individuality. We spend so much time trying to fit into a mold that we forget to celebrate the things that make us special.

Embracing imperfection is about accepting ourselves as

we are, flaws and all. It's about recognizing that our imperfections are not something to be ashamed of, but rather a source of strength, authenticity, and growth.

AUTHENTICITY: THE POWER OF BEING REAL

When we embrace our imperfections, we give ourselves permission to be authentic. We stop pretending to be someone we're not and start showing up in the world as our true selves. This authenticity is incredibly freeing. It allows us to connect with others on a deeper level, build genuine relationships, and express ourselves without fear of judgment.

Think about the people you admire most. Are they perfect? Probably not. In fact, it's often their flaws, their vulnerabilities, and their quirks that make them so relatable and endearing. When we embrace our own imperfections, we become more relatable, more approachable, and ultimately, more lovable.

LEARNING FROM MISTAKES: THE PATH TO GROWTH

Mistakes are not failures; they're opportunities for growth. When we make mistakes, we learn valuable lessons that we wouldn't have otherwise. We gain insights into our strengths and weaknesses, our values and priorities, and what truly matters to us.

Embracing imperfection means accepting that we're going to make mistakes along the way. It's about letting go of the need to be right all the time and instead focusing on learning and growing from our experiences. When we approach mistakes with curiosity and a willingness to learn, we open ourselves up to incredible personal development.

Think of a time when you made a mistake that led to a valuable lesson or a positive change in your life. Maybe it was a failed relationship that taught you what you truly value in a partner, a career misstep that led you to discover your true passion, or a personal setback that forced you to dig deep and find your inner strength.

These experiences, while often painful in the moment, can become powerful catalysts for growth. By embracing our imperfections and learning from our mistakes, we become more resilient, more adaptable, and better equipped to navigate the challenges life throws our way.

GROWTH: THE JOURNEY OF A LIFETIME

Embracing imperfection is a lifelong journey. It's about continuously challenging ourselves to step outside our comfort zones, to try new things, and to learn from our experiences. It's about letting go of the need for approval and validation from others and instead finding our own sense of self-worth and acceptance.

When we embrace imperfection, we open ourselves up to a world of possibilities. We become more creative, more resilient, and more open to new experiences. We stop comparing ourselves to others and start appreciating our own unique journey.

So, my friend, let go of the pressure to be perfect. Embrace your flaws, celebrate your quirks, and learn from your mistakes. You are perfectly imperfect, and that's what makes you beautiful.

EXERCISE: "PERFECTLY IMPERFECT" LIST

It's time to embrace your beautiful imperfections! Yes, you heard that right. We're going to celebrate those quirks, those flaws, those things you've been trying to hide or change. Why? Because those imperfections are what make you unique, interesting, and utterly human.

Think of it this way: Have you ever met someone who seemed too perfect? They always said the right thing, never made a mistake, and always looked flawless. Did you find them inspiring or intimidating? Relatable or robotic? Chances are, their "perfection" felt a bit... off.

That's because perfection doesn't exist. It's a myth we've been sold, a mirage that keeps us chasing an unattainable ideal. And in our relentless pursuit of perfection, we often miss out on the beauty and richness of our own unique imperfections.

YOUR PERFECTLY IMPERFECT LIST

Grab a pen and paper or open up a new document on your computer. Now, take a deep breath and start making a list of all the things you consider to be your imperfections or flaws. Don't hold back! Write down anything that comes to mind, no matter how big or small.

Here are some examples to get you started:

- *"I'm too sensitive."*
- *"I'm not good at public speaking."*
- *"I procrastinate."*
- *"I'm not as outgoing as I'd like to be."*
- *"I have a short temper."*
- *"I'm not very athletic."*

Take your time and really dig deep. Once you have a comprehensive list, it's time for the magic to happen.

REFRAMING YOUR IMPERFECTIONS

Now, go through your list and reframe each imperfection as a strength, a unique quality, or a potential for growth. Remember, the goal here isn't to deny or minimize your flaws; it's about seeing them in a new light.

Here are some examples of how you can reframe your imperfections:

- **"I'm too sensitive"** becomes "I'm deeply empathetic and compassionate."
- **"I'm not good at public speaking"** becomes "I'm a great listener and one-on-one communicator."
- **"I procrastinate"** becomes "I work best under pressure and can produce high-quality work in a short amount of time."
- **"I'm not as outgoing as I'd like to be"** becomes "I'm a thoughtful introvert who values deep connections."
- **"I have a short temper"** becomes "I'm passionate and I stand up for what I believe in."

- **"I'm not very athletic"** becomes "I have other talents and strengths that are equally valuable."

Notice how each reframe shifts the focus from a negative trait to a positive quality. Even the most challenging imperfections can be seen as opportunities for growth and self-improvement.

THE BEAUTY OF YOUR IMPERFECTIONS

By reframing your imperfections, you're not denying their existence. You're simply choosing to see them in a more empowering light. You're recognizing that your flaws don't define you; they are simply a part of who you are.

In fact, your imperfections are what make you unique and interesting. They are the spice that adds flavor to your life. They are the scars that tell your story. They are the challenges that have shaped you into the person you are today.

So, embrace your perfectly imperfect self. Love yourself for who you are, not who you think you should be. Celebrate your quirks, your flaws, and your unique way of being in the world. Because when you do, you'll discover that your imperfections are not weaknesses; they are your greatest strengths.

Day 23: Celebrate Your Strengths

Hey, superstar!

I know, I know. You're probably rolling your eyes at that. We're not used to being called "superstars," are we? We're more comfortable focusing on our flaws, our shortcomings, the areas where we feel we don't measure up.

But guess what? Today, we're changing that narrative. Today, we're flipping the script and putting the spotlight on something truly remarkable: your strengths.

Yes, *your* strengths. The unique talents, abilities, and qualities that make you, well, *you*. The things you do effortlessly, the things that light you up, the things that make you feel alive.

Why Celebrate Your Strengths?

Now, you might be thinking, "Why should I celebrate my strengths? Isn't it more important to focus on my weaknesses and improve those?"

While self-improvement is essential, it's equally important to recognize and appreciate the incredible gifts you already

possess. Focusing on your strengths doesn't mean ignoring your
areas for growth; it simply means shifting your focus from what you lack to what you already have.

Celebrating your strengths is a powerful way to:

- **Boost your confidence:** When you acknowledge your talents and abilities, you naturally feel more self-assured and capable.
- **Increase your motivation:** Focusing on your strengths can fuel your drive and enthusiasm for pursuing your goals.
- **Enhance your well-being:** Recognizing what you're good at can lead to greater happiness, satisfaction, and fulfillment.
- **Improve your performance:** When you play to your strengths, you're more likely to excel in your personal and professional life.

YOUR UNIQUE SUPERPOWERS

Remember those exercises we did earlier in the book, where you identified your passions, values, and talents? Those are your superpowers. They are the unique combination of qualities that make you stand out, the things that you bring to the table that no one else can.

Maybe you're a natural-born leader, with the ability to inspire and motivate others. Or perhaps you're a creative genius, with a knack for expressing yourself through art, music, or writing. Maybe you're a problem-solver, a peacemaker, a caregiver, or a teacher.

Whatever your strengths may be, they are valuable. They are your gifts to the world, and it's time to start celebrating them.

EXERCISE: STRENGTHS SHOWCASE

Ready to step into the spotlight? Today's exercise is all about showcasing your strengths.

Choose one of your strengths that you feel particularly proud of. It could be a skill you've honed, a talent you were born with, or a quality that others admire in you.

Then, find a way to share this strength with someone else. You could:

- **Teach someone a skill:** If you're a whiz at cooking, offer to teach a friend a new recipe.
- **Offer a helping hand:** If you're a great listener, lend an ear to someone who needs to talk.
- **Express your talent:** If you're a talented artist, share your work with others.

By sharing your strengths, you not only benefit others but also reinforce your own sense of self-worth and confidence. It's a win-win situation!

Remember, your strengths are not meant to be hidden away. They are meant to be celebrated, shared, and used to make a positive impact on the world. So go out there and shine, superstar!

IDENTIFYING YOUR STRENGTHS

Remember those superpowers you uncovered back in [Chapter Reference]? The unique talents, skills, and qualities that make you, well, *you*? It's time to dust them off and give them a standing ovation, because they hold the key to unlocking your full potential.

Let's face it, we've all been conditioned to focus on our weaknesses. From school report cards that highlighted areas for improvement to well-meaning friends who pointed out our flaws, it's easy to get caught up in the "fix-it" mentality. We spend countless hours trying to improve the things we're not naturally good at, hoping to become a well-rounded jack-of-all-trades.

But here's the thing: trying to be good at everything is a recipe for exhaustion and mediocrity. When we spread ourselves too thin, we dilute our energy and focus. We become a watered-down version of ourselves, never fully tapping into our true potential.

The alternative? Embrace your superpowers!

Think of your strengths as your personal arsenal of tools, each one uniquely designed to help you thrive. Maybe you're a natural problem-solver, a creative visionary, a compassionate listener, or a charismatic leader. Whatever your strengths may be, they are the foundation of your success and fulfillment.

When you focus on your strengths, amazing things happen:

- **Increased Confidence:** When you're doing what you're naturally good at, you feel more competent, capable, and confident. This boost in self-assurance allows you to take on challenges, pursue your dreams, and achieve your goals.

- **Enhanced Motivation:** When you're engaged in activities that utilize your strengths, you're more likely to feel energized, enthusiastic, and motivated. You become intrinsically driven to excel, simply because you enjoy the process.
- **Greater Success:** Focusing on your strengths allows you to leverage your natural talents and abilities, leading to higher levels of performance and achievement. You're more likely to succeed in your endeavors when you're playing to your strengths.
- **Deeper Fulfillment:** When you're using your strengths in a way that aligns with your values and purpose, you experience a profound sense of fulfillment. You feel like you're making a meaningful contribution and living a life that is true to yourself.

This doesn't mean you should ignore your weaknesses altogether. We all have areas where we can improve and grow. But instead of obsessing over your shortcomings, try reframing them as areas for potential growth. For example, if you're not naturally organized, you can learn strategies and systems to compensate for that weakness.

By focusing on your strengths, you free yourself from the trap of comparison and self-doubt. You stop trying to fit into someone else's mold and start celebrating your unique talents and abilities. You become more authentic, more confident, and more empowered to create a life that is truly fulfilling.

Remember, your strengths are not just about what you're

good at; they're also about who you are at your core. They reflect your values, passions, and purpose. By embracing and utilizing your strengths, you not only achieve greater success but also live a life that is more meaningful, authentic, and joyful.

So, take a moment to revisit the strengths you identified earlier in this book. How can you start incorporating them more intentionally into your daily life? What are some ways you can use your superpowers to make a difference in the world?

As you continue on your journey of self-discovery and purpose, remember that your strengths are your greatest assets. Embrace them, celebrate them, and use them to create a life that you truly love.

USING YOUR STRENGTHS FOR GOOD

Now that you've taken the time to rediscover and appreciate your unique strengths, it's time to unleash them on the world! But not just for personal gain – let's aim higher. Let's talk about how you can use your strengths to make a real difference in the lives of others.

THE POWER OF SHARING YOUR GIFTS

Think about it this way: Your strengths aren't just random traits.

They're your superpowers, the special tools you've been given to contribute to the world. When you use your strengths in service to others, you're not only making a positive impact on their lives, but you're also tapping into a deeper sense of purpose and fulfillment for yourself.

Maybe you're a natural-born listener. Could you use that strength to volunteer at a crisis hotline, offer a supportive ear to a friend in need, or even create a podcast that offers guidance and encouragement to others?

Perhaps you're a creative problem-solver. Could you use your ingenuity to tackle a community issue, develop innovative solutions for your workplace, or even just help a neighbor troubleshoot a DIY project?

Even the smallest actions, when fueled by your strengths, can create a ripple effect of positive change.

UNLEASHING YOUR STRENGTHS IN EVERYDAY LIFE

You don't have to quit your job or start a nonprofit to make a difference. There are countless ways to integrate your strengths into your everyday life:

- **At Work:** Look for opportunities to utilize your strengths within your current role. If you're a skilled communicator, maybe you could take on a leadership position or mentor a new employee. If you're a detail-oriented person, perhaps you could streamline a process or develop a more efficient system.
- **In Your Hobbies:** If you love to write, you could share your stories and insights with others through a blog or volunteer to write for a local organization. If you're passionate about fitness, you could lead a community

exercise group or mentor someone on their health journey.
- **In Your Relationships:** Use your strengths to nurture and support your loved ones. If you're a compassionate person, offer a listening ear and a shoulder to lean on. If you're a natural comedian, bring laughter and joy into your relationships.

FINDING YOUR NICHE

Take some time to reflect on how your strengths align with your passions and values. What causes are you passionate about? What problems in the world would you like to help solve? How can your unique talents contribute to making a difference?

Don't be afraid to experiment. Try volunteering for different organizations, exploring new hobbies, or offering your skills to friends and family. As you start using your strengths in service of others, you'll gain a deeper understanding of your purpose and how you can best contribute to the world.

OVERCOMING OBSTACLES

Of course, there may be times when self-doubt creeps in or you face obstacles along the way. Remember, it's okay to feel unsure or hesitant at times. But don't let fear hold you back from sharing your gifts with the world.

Use the tools you've learned throughout this book to manage your self-doubt, reframe negative thoughts, and build your confidence. Remind yourself of the positive impact you can make and the joy that comes from using your strengths for good.

Remember, you don't have to do it alone. Seek support from loved ones, mentors, or coaches who can encourage and guide you on your journey. Join communities of like-minded individuals who share your passions and values. Surround yourself with people who believe in you and your ability to make a difference.

THE RIPPLE EFFECT OF GIVING

When you use your strengths for good, you not only benefit others, but you also create a ripple effect of positivity that spreads throughout your community and beyond. Your actions can inspire others to do the same, creating a chain reaction of kindness, compassion, and generosity.

By sharing your unique gifts with the world, you're not just making a difference; you're also living a more meaningful, fulfilling life. You're tapping into your purpose, expressing your authentic self, and creating a legacy that will last long after you're gone.

EXERCISE: STRENGTHS SHOWCASE

You've spent the last few weeks delving deep into your passions, values, and purpose. You've identified your "why" and started taking steps to align your actions with your goals. Now,

it's time to shine a light on your unique strengths and share your brilliance with the world.

Think back to the strengths and talents you identified earlier in this journey. Remember that feeling of pride and excitement when you realized just how much you have to offer? It's time to tap into that energy and let your strengths take center stage.

WHY SHARE YOUR STRENGTHS?

Sharing your strengths isn't about bragging or showing off. It's about recognizing the unique gifts you possess and using them to make a positive impact on others. When you share your strengths, you not only benefit those around you but also strengthen your own sense of purpose and self-worth.

Research shows that using our strengths regularly can lead to increased happiness, engagement, and productivity. It can also help us build stronger relationships, enhance our creativity, and even improve our physical health. So, sharing your strengths isn't just a nice thing to do—it's essential for your overall well-being.

HOW TO SHARE YOUR STRENGTHS

There are countless ways to share your strengths with others. Here are a few ideas to get you started:

- **Teach Someone a Skill:** Do you have a knack for baking, coding, or playing an instrument? Offer to teach a friend, family member, or coworker. Sharing your knowledge not only helps them but also reinforces your own mastery.

- **Offer a Helping Hand:** Are you a great listener, organizer, or problem-solver? Look for opportunities to help someone in need. This could be as simple as offering a listening ear to a friend who's going through a tough time or helping a colleague organize a project.
- **Express a Talent:** Do you have a creative talent, such as writing, painting, or singing? Share your work with others. This could involve performing at an open mic night, submitting your writing to a publication, or simply showing your art to a friend.
- **Mentor Someone:** Are you experienced in a particular field? Offer to mentor someone who's just starting out. Sharing your knowledge and expertise can be incredibly rewarding for both you and your mentee.
- **Volunteer Your Time:** Find a cause you care about and volunteer your skills and talents. This could involve tutoring students, helping at an animal shelter, or organizing a community event.

THE STRENGTH SHOWCASE CHALLENGE

This week, I challenge you to share one of your strengths with someone else. Choose an action that feels authentic and meaningful to you. It doesn't have to be a grand gesture – even small acts of kindness can have a big impact.

Here are some additional tips for completing the Strength Showcase Challenge:

- **Start Small:** If you're feeling hesitant, start with a small, low-pressure activity. Offer to help a friend with

a task they're struggling with or share a creative project you've been working on.
- **Be Specific:** When sharing your strength, be specific about what you offer. Instead of saying, "I'm good at writing," say, "I'd love to help you edit your resume" or "I'd be happy to give you feedback on your blog post."
- **Don't Underestimate Yourself:** We often downplay our strengths or assume that others won't find them valuable. Remember, your unique skills and talents have the power to make a real difference in someone's life.
- **Embrace the Experience:** Sharing your strengths can be a vulnerable experience, but it's also incredibly rewarding. Embrace the opportunity to connect with others, make a positive impact, and strengthen your own sense of purpose.

By participating in the Strength Showcase Challenge, you'll not only brighten someone else's day but also reinforce your own belief in your abilities. You'll experience the joy of giving back, the satisfaction of using your talents, and the fulfillment of living a life that is aligned with your purpose.

Day 24: Cultivate Gratitude

Have you ever noticed how, on some days, everything seems to go wrong? You spill coffee on your shirt, miss the bus, and get stuck in traffic. By the time you finally arrive at work, you're already stressed and grumpy, convinced the entire universe is conspiring against you.

But then there are those other days when, even if a few things go awry, you somehow maintain a sense of peace and optimism. You laugh off the coffee stain, find an alternate route to work, and use the extra time in traffic to listen to an inspiring podcast. What's the difference between these two scenarios?

The answer, my friend, is gratitude.

Gratitude is the simple yet profound act of acknowledging and appreciating the good things in our lives. It's about shifting our focus from what we lack to what we have, from what's wrong to what's right. And it's a powerful tool for cultivating joy, resilience, and a more positive outlook on life.

In this chapter, we'll delve deeper into the transformative power of gratitude. We'll explore how it can help us:

- **Reduce stress and anxiety:** When we focus on what we're grateful for, it's harder to get bogged down by worry and negativity. Gratitude activates the calming parasympathetic nervous system, helping us to feel more relaxed and at ease.
- **Boost happiness and well-being:** Studies have shown that practicing gratitude can significantly increase our happiness levels. It helps us savor positive experiences, cultivate joy, and build a more optimistic outlook on life.
- **Strengthen relationships:** Expressing gratitude to others strengthens our bonds, fosters a sense of connection, and deepens our appreciation for the people in our lives.
- **Improve physical health:** Gratitude has been linked to better sleep, lower blood pressure, and a stronger immune system. It can even help reduce pain and improve recovery from illness.
- **Build resilience:** When we cultivate gratitude, we develop a greater capacity to cope with challenges and setbacks. We learn to find silver linings, focus on solutions, and bounce back from adversity.

But gratitude is not just about feeling good; it's about a fundamental shift in perspective. It's about recognizing the abundance that already exists in our lives, even when things are tough. It's about appreciating the small joys, the everyday miracles, and the people who enrich our lives.

In the following sections, we'll explore how to make

gratitude a way of life, not just a fleeting feeling. We'll discuss practical
ways to cultivate gratitude every day, even when it feels challenging. And we'll provide you with exercises and prompts to help you deepen your gratitude practice and reap its many benefits.

GRATITUDE BEYOND THE JOURNAL

While gratitude journaling is a powerful tool for cultivating thankfulness, it's just the tip of the iceberg. Gratitude isn't meant to be confined to the pages of a notebook; it's a way of life, a lens through which we can view the world with greater appreciation and joy.

Think of gratitude as a muscle. The more you use it, the stronger it becomes. And just like any muscle, it needs to be exercised regularly to maintain its strength and flexibility. Journaling is like a focused workout for your gratitude muscle, but there are countless ways to flex it throughout your day, weaving thankfulness into the fabric of your life.

EXPRESSING APPRECIATION: THE GIFT OF ACKNOWLEDGMENT

One of the simplest and most powerful ways to practice gratitude is by expressing appreciation to others. When someone does something kind for you, big or small, take a moment to acknowledge it. Say "thank you" with sincerity, send a handwritten note, or offer a genuine compliment. Let people know that you value their presence in your life and that you appreciate their contributions.

Expressing gratitude isn't just about being polite; it's about fostering connection, deepening relationships, and creating a positive ripple effect. When you express appreciation, you not only uplift the person you're thanking but also boost your own happiness and well-being. It's a win-win situation!

SAVORING POSITIVE EXPERIENCES: THE ART OF MINDFULNESS

In our fast-paced world, it's easy to rush through life without truly appreciating the positive moments. We might achieve a goal, experience a beautiful sunset, or share a laugh with a loved one, but then quickly move on to the next thing without fully savoring the experience.

Practicing gratitude involves slowing down and intentionally focusing on the good things in our lives. Take a moment to pause and appreciate the taste of your morning coffee, the warmth of the sun on your skin, or the sound of your child's laughter. Notice the details, the sensations, the emotions. By savoring positive experiences, we amplify their impact and create lasting memories that nourish our souls.

NOTICING BEAUTY: OPENING YOUR EYES TO THE EXTRAORDINARY

Gratitude isn't just about appreciating the big events or milestones in our lives; it's about finding beauty and wonder in the everyday. It's about noticing the intricate patterns of a flower, the vibrant colors of a sunset, the kindness of a stranger.

When we cultivate a sense of awe and appreciation for the world around us, we open ourselves up to a deeper level of gratitude. We realize that even the most mundane moments can be filled with extraordinary beauty and meaning.

GRATITUDE IN ACTION: MAKING A DIFFERENCE

Gratitude is more than just a feeling; it's a call to action. When we feel grateful for the blessings in our lives, we're naturally inspired to give back and make a positive contribution to the world.

This could involve volunteering your time, donating to a cause you care about, or simply offering a helping hand to someone in need. By expressing your gratitude through action, you not only reinforce the positive emotions you're feeling but also create a ripple effect of kindness and generosity.

THE RIPPLE EFFECT OF GRATITUDE

Gratitude is contagious. When you express appreciation to others, savor positive experiences, and notice the beauty around you, you create a ripple effect that extends far beyond yourself.

Your gratitude can inspire others to do the same, creating a more positive and supportive environment for everyone. It can also strengthen your relationships, improve your mental and physical health, and increase your overall happiness and well-being.

GRATITUDE: A WAY OF LIFE

Remember, gratitude is not a one-time event; it's a way of life. It's a conscious choice to focus on the good, to appreciate the present moment, and to express our thanks for the blessings in our lives.

By weaving gratitude into your everyday routine, you'll discover a newfound sense of joy, resilience, and connection. You'll learn to appreciate the simple pleasures, navigate challenges with grace, and live a life that is rich with meaning and purpose.

So go forth and express your gratitude! Say thank you, savor the moment, and notice the beauty around you. Let gratitude be your guiding light, illuminating your path towards a happier, healthier, and more fulfilling life.

THE RIPPLE EFFECT OF GRATITUDE

Gratitude isn't just a warm, fuzzy feeling you get when someone does something nice. It's a powerful force that can transform your life, your relationships, and even your community. Think of it like a pebble tossed into a still pond, creating ripples that spread outward, touching everything in their path.

GRATITUDE'S PERSONAL TOUCH:

When you make gratitude a habit, it's like giving yourself a daily dose of emotional vitamins. Research has shown that gratitude can:

- **Boost your happiness:** Gratitude rewires your brain to focus on the positive, making you feel more content and joyful.
- **Reduce stress and anxiety:** Focusing on what you're thankful for helps to counteract stress hormones, leaving you feeling calmer and more at ease.
- **Improve your sleep:** Gratitude journaling before bed has been linked to better sleep quality and duration.
- **Strengthen your immune system:** Studies suggest that grateful people tend to get sick less often and recover faster.
- **Increase your resilience:** When you practice gratitude, you're better equipped to handle challenges and bounce back from setbacks.

But gratitude's benefits go far beyond your own well-being. It has a ripple effect that extends to the people around you.

GRATITUDE'S RELATIONAL REACH:

When you express gratitude to others, you create a positive feedback loop that strengthens your bonds and deepens your connection. Here's how:

- **Stronger relationships:** Expressing gratitude to your loved ones, friends, colleagues, or even strangers, fosters feelings of appreciation, warmth, and goodwill. It strengthens your existing bonds and helps to build new ones.
- **Improved communication:** When you practice gratitude, you become more attuned to the positive qualities in others and are more likely to express your appreciation for them. This creates a more open and positive communication dynamic.
- **Increased empathy and understanding:** Gratitude encourages you to see the world through the eyes of others, fostering empathy and understanding. This can lead to deeper, more meaningful relationships.
- **More generosity and kindness:** Grateful people are more likely to help others, volunteer their time, and perform acts of kindness. This creates a ripple effect of generosity and compassion.
- **Enhanced conflict resolution:** Gratitude can help to de-escalate conflicts and find solutions more quickly. When you're focused on the positive aspects of your relationship, it's easier to find common ground and resolve disagreements.

Imagine the impact of a simple "thank you" or a heartfelt note of appreciation. It can brighten someone's day, boost their self-esteem, and inspire them to pay it forward.

Gratitude's Community Impact:

The ripple effect of gratitude doesn't stop at your personal relationships. It extends to the broader community, creating a more positive and supportive environment for everyone.

- **Stronger communities:** When gratitude is practiced on a wider scale, it can lead to increased trust, cooperation, and social cohesion. It can inspire people to work together to solve problems and create positive change.
- **Increased civic engagement:** Grateful individuals are more likely to participate in community activities, volunteer their time, and vote in elections. This can lead to a more engaged and responsive citizenry.
- **Improved mental health outcomes:** Research suggests that gratitude can reduce symptoms of depression and anxiety, not just on an individual level, but also on a community level.
- **Reduced social isolation:** When people express gratitude and appreciation for each other, it creates a sense of belonging and connection, reducing feelings of isolation and loneliness.
- **A more positive social climate:** Gratitude fosters a culture of appreciation, respect, and kindness. This can lead to a more positive and supportive social environment for everyone.

When we express gratitude for the contributions of others, whether it's a police officer, a teacher, a healthcare worker, or a local volunteer, we uplift their spirits and reinforce their sense of purpose. This creates a positive cycle of appreciation and contribution that benefits the entire community.

Gratitude is not just a feeling; it's a way of life. It's a

conscious choice to focus on the good, to appreciate the blessings in our lives, and to express our thanks to those around us. When we practice gratitude, we not only improve our own well-being, but we also create a ripple effect of positivity that transforms our relationships, strengthens our communities, and makes the world a better place.

EXERCISE: GRATITUDE LETTER

Remember that teacher who believed in you when no one else did? The friend who always had your back, no matter what? The
mentor who guided you through a difficult time? Or maybe it's your partner, your parent, or even a stranger whose kindness touched your heart.

Today, you're going to express your gratitude to this special person by writing them a heartfelt letter. Don't worry, this isn't about perfect grammar or fancy words. It's about genuine appreciation and acknowledging the impact they've had on your life.

WHY WRITE A GRATITUDE LETTER?

- Gratitude is a powerful emotion that can transform your perspective and enhance your well-being.
- Expressing gratitude strengthens relationships and deepens connections.
- Writing a letter allows you to reflect on the positive influences in your life and express your emotions in a thoughtful way.

Getting Started

1. **Choose Your Recipient:** Think about someone who has made a significant positive impact on your life. It could be someone you know well or someone you haven't seen in years.
2. **Set the Mood:** Find a quiet space where you won't be interrupted. Light a candle, put on some calming music, or do whatever helps you relax and focus.
3. **Gather Your Thoughts:** Take a few minutes to reflect on the specific ways this person has influenced you. What qualities do you admire in them? What specific actions or words have made a difference in your life? Jot down some notes to help you organize your thoughts.

WRITING YOUR LETTER

- **Dear [Recipient's Name]:** Start your letter with a warm salutation.
- **Express Your Gratitude:** Begin by expressing your sincere gratitude for their presence in your life. Let them know how much you appreciate their support, guidance, kindness, or any other qualities that have positively impacted you.
- **Share Specific Examples:** Don't just say "thank you." Go deeper and share specific examples of how this person has influenced you. Did they offer encouragement when you were feeling down? Did they teach you a valuable skill? Did they simply listen with compassion

and understanding? The more specific you can be, the more meaningful your letter will be.

- **Acknowledge Their Impact:** Explain how their actions or words have made a difference in your life. Have they helped you overcome a challenge? Have they inspired you to pursue your dreams? Have they simply made your life brighter and more joyful?
- **Express Your Wishes for Them:** Close your letter by expressing your best wishes for their happiness, health, and continued success. Let them know that you are grateful for their presence in your life and that you hope to stay connected with them in the future.
- **Sincerely, [Your Name]:** Sign your letter with a warm closing.

ADDITIONAL TIPS:

- **Be Authentic:** Write from the heart and use your own words. Don't worry about sounding perfect or poetic.
- **Be Specific:** The more specific you can be about the impact this person has had on your life, the more meaningful your letter will be.
- **Focus on the Positive:** Even if your relationship with this person has had its ups and downs, focus on the positive aspects and the ways they have enriched your life.
- **Don't Overthink It:** The most important thing is to express your gratitude. Don't get bogged down in trying to write the perfect letter.
- **Deliver Your Letter:** Once you've finished your letter, consider delivering it in person, mailing it, or sending

it electronically. The act of sharing your gratitude will not only brighten their day but also deepen your connection with them.

Example of a Gratitude Letter:

Dear [Mentor's Name],

I'm writing to express my deepest gratitude for your unwavering support and guidance throughout my career. Your belief in me, even when I doubted myself, has been a constant source of inspiration.

I'll never forget the time when I was struggling with a difficult project. You not only offered practical advice but also reminded me of my strengths and encouraged me to persevere. Your words gave me the confidence I needed to push through and ultimately achieve success.

Thank you for always being willing to lend a listening ear, offer constructive feedback, and celebrate my achievements. Your mentorship has been invaluable to my personal and professional growth.

I am so grateful to have you in my life. I wish you all the best in your own endeavors.

Sincerely,

[Your Name]

Go Forth and Give Thanks:

The act of writing a gratitude letter is a gift, both to the recipient and to yourself. It's a way to deepen connections, foster positivity, and remind ourselves of the blessings in our lives. So, take the time to express your gratitude today. You'll be glad you did.

Day 25: Practice Self-Compassion

Imagine this: Your best friend comes to you, distraught after a major setback. Maybe they lost a job, ended a relationship, or made a decision they deeply regret. How would you respond?

You wouldn't berate them, call them names, or tell them they're worthless. You'd offer a listening ear, a warm embrace, and words of encouragement. You'd remind them of their strengths, their resilience, and their capacity for growth. You'd be their biggest cheerleader, even when they couldn't cheer for themselves.

Now, imagine extending that same kindness and compassion to yourself. That, my friend, is the essence of self-compassion.

THE INNER CRITIC VS. THE INNER BFF

We all have an inner critic—that nagging voice that tells us we're not good enough, smart enough, or worthy enough. It whispers doubts, magnifies our flaws, and berates us for our mistakes. This inner critic can be relentless, especially when we're feeling vulnerable or down.

But what if we could replace that inner critic with an inner BFF—a voice that offers unconditional love, support, and understanding? A voice that reminds us that we're human, that we're doing the best we can, and that we deserve kindness and compassion, especially from ourselves.

That's where self-compassion comes in. It's about treating ourselves with the same care and concern that we would offer to a dear friend. It's about recognizing our own suffering and responding with warmth, understanding, and a desire to alleviate our pain.

THE SCIENCE OF SELF-COMPASSION

Self-compassion isn't just a feel-good concept; it's backed by science. Research shows that practicing self-compassion can lead to a wide range of benefits, including:

- **Reduced stress and anxiety:** Self-compassion helps us manage difficult emotions without getting overwhelmed.
- **Increased resilience:** It helps us bounce back from setbacks and challenges with greater ease.
- **Improved relationships:** When we're kind to ourselves, we're more likely to be kind to others.
- **Greater happiness and well-being:** Self-compassion cultivates a sense of inner peace and contentment.

In fact, studies have shown that self-compassion is a

stronger predictor of happiness than self-esteem. This is because self-esteem is often based on external validation and comparison to others, while self-compassion is rooted in an unconditional acceptance of ourselves, flaws and all.

THE POWER OF SELF-COMPASSION

Self-compassion is not about self-indulgence or letting ourselves off the hook. It's not about ignoring our flaws or pretending that everything is okay when it's not.

Instead, self-compassion is about acknowledging our struggles with kindness and understanding. It's about recognizing that we are all human, that we all make mistakes, and that we all deserve love and compassion.

When we practice self-compassion, we create a safe space within ourselves to heal, grow, and thrive. We become our own best friend, our own source of strength and support. And that, my friend, is a truly liberating feeling.

WHAT IS SELF-COMPASSION?

Imagine this: You've messed up. You made a mistake, dropped the ball, or simply didn't live up to your own expectations. Maybe you missed a deadline at work, said something hurtful to a loved one, or made a financial blunder. Your first instinct might be to berate yourself, replay the scenario over and over in your mind, and criticize your every move.

Sound familiar? We've all been there. It's that harsh inner voice that tells us we're not good enough, smart enough, or capable enough. It's that relentless self-judgment that can leave us feeling deflated, ashamed, and paralyzed by fear.

But what if there was a different way to respond to these inevitable setbacks and imperfections? What if, instead of beating yourself up, you could offer yourself kindness, understanding, and forgiveness?

That's where self-compassion comes in.

SELF-COMPASSION: YOUR INNER ALLY

Self-compassion is not about self-indulgence or letting yourself off the hook. It's not about ignoring your shortcomings or pretending everything is okay when it's not.

Instead, self-compassion is about treating yourself with the same kindness, care, and concern that you would offer to a good friend who is going through a tough time. It's about acknowledging your pain and suffering without judgment, recognizing that you're human and imperfect, and offering yourself support and encouragement.

Think of it as having your own personal cheerleader on the sidelines of your life, reminding you that you're worthy, capable, and deserving of love and respect, even when you stumble or fall.

THE THREE COMPONENTS OF SELF-COMPASSION

Self-compassion consists of three key components:

1. **Self-Kindness vs. Self-Judgment:** This means treating

yourself with warmth and understanding rather than harsh criticism. It's about being gentle with yourself when you're struggling, rather than adding fuel to the fire of self-flagellation.
2. **Common Humanity vs. Isolation:** This involves recognizing that everyone makes mistakes, experiences setbacks, and feels inadequate at times. It's about understanding that suffering is part of the shared human experience, not a sign that you're flawed or alone.
3. **Mindfulness vs. Over-Identification:** This refers to being aware of your thoughts and emotions without becoming overwhelmed by them. It's about observing your feelings with curiosity and acceptance, rather than getting swept away by negativity or self-pity.

WHY SELF-COMPASSION MATTERS

Practicing self-compassion has a profound impact on our well-being and our ability to thrive in life. Research shows that self-compassion is linked to:

- **Reduced stress and anxiety:** Self-compassion helps us manage difficult emotions without getting overwhelmed by them.
- **Increased resilience:** When we're kind to ourselves, we're better able to bounce back from setbacks and challenges.
- **Improved relationships:** Self-compassion allows us to be more understanding and empathetic towards others.
- **Enhanced motivation:** When we believe in ourselves

and our ability to learn and grow, we're more likely to take on new challenges and pursue our goals.
- **Greater happiness and well-being:** Self-compassion fosters a sense of inner peace, contentment, and self-worth.

In essence, self-compassion is a superpower that can help us navigate life's ups and downs with greater ease and resilience. It's a key ingredient in creating a life of purpose, passion, and no regrets.

In the next section, we'll explore some practical ways to cultivate self-compassion in your daily life. Get ready to discover your inner ally and unlock the power of kindness towards yourself.

SELF-COMPASSION VS. SELF-PITY

Okay, friend, let's talk about two emotions that often get confused: self-compassion and self-pity. These two feelings might seem similar on the surface, but they couldn't be more different in their impact on your life. Think of them like two different GPS systems. One guides you towards a destination of healing and growth, while the other keeps you circling in a roundabout of negativity and despair.

SELF-PITY: THE EMOTIONAL ROUNDABOUT

Ever found yourself wallowing in a pool of "poor me"? That's self-pity at work. It's a tempting trap, especially when life throws us curveballs. Self-pity tells us we're victims, that we're the only ones suffering, and that nothing will ever get better. It thrives on isolation, magnifying our problems and minimizing our strengths.

Think of it like this: you're driving down the road of life, and self-pity is that GPS voice that keeps saying, "Rerouting, rerouting," every time you hit a bump. It keeps you circling in the same negative thoughts, making you feel helpless and hopeless.

Self-pity might provide temporary comfort, but it's a dead end. It drains your energy, prevents you from taking action, and ultimately keeps you stuck. It's like hitting the snooze button on your dreams and settling for a life of mediocrity and discontent.

SELF-COMPASSION: YOUR GPS TO GROWTH

Now, let's switch to a different GPS—self-compassion. This is the voice that says, "I see you're struggling, but I'm here with you. Let's figure this out together." Self-compassion acknowledges our pain and suffering without judgment. It reminds us that we're human, that we make mistakes, and that setbacks are a natural part of life.

Self-compassion is like having a supportive friend who offers a listening ear, a warm hug, and a gentle nudge in the right direction. It doesn't deny our pain; it embraces it with kindness and understanding. It reminds us that we're not alone in our struggles and that we have the strength and resilience to overcome them.

When we practice self-compassion, we create a safe space within ourselves to heal and grow. We become more resilient in the face of challenges, more accepting of our imperfections, and more open to new possibilities. We move from a victim mindset

to an empowered mindset, taking responsibility for our lives and making choices that align with our values and goals.

THE DIFFERENCE THAT MAKES ALL THE DIFFERENCE

Here's a quick comparison to help you distinguish between self-pity and self-compassion:

Self-Pity	Self-Compassion
Focuses on the problem	Focuses on the solution
Magnifies suffering	Acknowledges suffering
Isolates and separates	Connects and unites
Blames self and others	Offers understanding and forgiveness
Leads to inaction and despair	Leads to action and hope
Feels like a dead end	Feels like a new beginning

NAVIGATING YOUR EMOTIONS

So, how do you cultivate self-compassion and avoid the trap of self-pity? It starts with awareness. Notice when you're falling into negative self-talk and catastrophizing. Instead of berating yourself, try offering yourself kind words and encouragement, just as you would to a friend in need.

Remember, you're not alone in this. Everyone experiences setbacks, failures, and disappointments. But it's how we respond to those challenges that define our character and determine our path. By choosing self-compassion over self-pity, you're choosing a path of healing, growth, and ultimately, a regret-free life.

So next time you find yourself at an emotional crossroads, ask yourself, "Which GPS am I following?" Choose the one that leads you towards your purpose, your dreams, and your most authentic self. Choose self-compassion.

EXERCISE: SELF-COMPASSION BREAK

Remember that friend who always knows just what to say when you're feeling down? The one who listens without judgment, offers a warm hug, and reminds you of your strengths? Today, I want you to become that friend for yourself.

Life isn't always sunshine and rainbows. We all face challenges, setbacks, and moments of self-doubt. It's during these tough times that self-compassion becomes our lifeline. Instead of beating ourselves up, we learn to offer ourselves the same kindness and understanding we would extend to a dear friend.

WHAT IS SELF-COMPASSION?

Self-compassion isn't about self-pity or making excuses

for our shortcomings. It's about recognizing our own suffering and responding with care and understanding. It's about acknowledging that we're human, and that making mistakes and experiencing pain is part of the human experience.

The Self-Compassion Break is a simple yet powerful tool you can use anytime you're feeling overwhelmed, stressed, or self-critical. It's a way to pause, reconnect with your inner wisdom, and offer yourself the support you need to move through difficult emotions.

How to Take a Self-Compassion Break

1. **Notice and Acknowledge:** The first step is to simply notice what you're feeling. What emotions are present? Are you feeling stressed, sad, angry, frustrated? Name the emotion without judgment. Say to yourself, "This is a moment of suffering."
2. **Connect to Your Humanity:** Remind yourself that you're not alone in your suffering. Everyone experiences pain, disappointment, and setbacks. Say to yourself, "Suffering is a part of life" or "I'm not alone in this."
3. **Offer Yourself Kindness:** Place your hand on your heart or any other place on your body that feels comforting. Take a few deep breaths and offer yourself words of kindness and encouragement. You might say, "May I be kind to myself," "May I be patient," or "May I forgive myself."

ADDITIONAL PHRASES FOR YOUR SELF-COMPASSION BREAK

- *"This is a tough moment, but I can handle it."*
- *"May I be strong and find a way through this."*
- *"I am worthy of love and compassion, even when I struggle."*
- *"May I accept myself as I am, with all my flaws and imperfections."*

TIPS FOR PRACTICING SELF-COMPASSION:

- **Be patient:** Self-compassion takes practice. Don't get discouraged if it feels awkward or unfamiliar at first. Keep practicing, and it will become more natural over time.
- **Be kind to yourself:** Treat yourself with the same kindness and understanding you would offer to a dear friend.
- **Validate your feelings:** Don't try to dismiss or minimize your emotions. Acknowledge them and allow yourself to feel them fully.
- **Remember your humanity:** Remind yourself that you're not perfect, and that's okay. We all make mistakes and experience setbacks.
- **Focus on the present:** When you're caught in a spiral of self-criticism, bring yourself back to the present moment. Focus on your breath or your senses.
- **Seek support:** If you're struggling with self-compassion,

don't hesitate to reach out to a trusted friend, family member, therapist, or coach for support.

THE BENEFITS OF SELF-COMPASSION

Practicing self-compassion has been shown to have a wide range of benefits, including:

- **Reduced stress and anxiety:** Self-compassion can help us manage stress and anxiety by activating our soothing system and calming our nervous system.
- **Increased happiness and well-being:** Studies have shown that self-compassion is linked to greater happiness, life satisfaction, and optimism.
- **Improved relationships:** When we're kind to ourselves, we're more likely to be kind to others, leading to healthier and more fulfilling relationships.
- **Increased resilience:** Self-compassion helps us bounce back from setbacks and challenges more quickly.
- **Reduced self-criticism and shame:** By treating ourselves with understanding and kindness, we can break free from the cycle of self-criticism and shame.

INTEGRATING SELF-COMPASSION INTO YOUR LIFE

Self-compassion is not a one-time fix; it's an ongoing practice. Make it a habit to incorporate self-compassion breaks into your daily routine, especially during times of stress or difficulty. You can also try practicing self-compassion during other activities, such as mindful walking, yoga, or journaling.

Remember, self-compassion is a gift you give yourself. It's a way to nurture your emotional well-being, build resilience, and create a more positive and fulfilling life. So be kind to yourself, my friend. You deserve it.

Day 26: Connect with Others

Let's be real for a moment: We weren't meant to do this life alone. As humans, we are inherently social creatures, wired for connection. Yet, in our quest for independence and self-reliance, we can sometimes forget the profound impact that meaningful relationships have on our well-being and our ability to thrive.

Think about it. Who are the people you turn to when you're facing a challenge, celebrating a victory, or simply need a listening ear? Who makes you laugh until your sides hurt, challenges you to grow, or inspires you to be a better version of yourself?

These are the people who make life richer, more vibrant, and more meaningful. They are our cheerleaders, our confidants, our partners in crime, and our pillars of support. They remind us that we are not alone in this journey, and that we are stronger together than we are apart.

THE POWER OF CONNECTION IN OVERCOMING FEAR AND REGRET

When we're feeling stuck in fear or consumed by regret, it can be tempting to isolate ourselves. We may feel ashamed,

unworthy, or afraid of being judged by others. But this isolation only deepens our pain and keeps us trapped in a cycle of negativity.

Connecting with others, on the other hand, can be a powerful antidote to fear and regret. Sharing our struggles with trusted friends or family members can help us feel less alone, gain new perspectives, and find solutions we might not have seen on our own.

Supportive relationships can also help us build resilience and self-esteem. When we know we have people who believe in us and are rooting for our success, we're more likely to take risks, pursue our dreams, and overcome challenges. And when we inevitably stumble or make mistakes, those same people can offer compassion, encouragement, and a helping hand.

BUILDING MEANINGFUL CONNECTIONS

In today's fast-paced, technology-driven world, it can be challenging to cultivate genuine connections. We may be surrounded by people but feel disconnected from them. We may have hundreds of social media "friends" but lack deep, meaningful relationships.

This is where intentionality comes in. Building meaningful connections requires effort, vulnerability, and a willingness to invest time and energy in cultivating relationships. It means being present for others, listening with empathy, offering support, and showing genuine interest in their lives.

It also means being willing to be vulnerable ourselves. Sharing our struggles, fears, and hopes with others creates a deeper level of intimacy and trust. It allows us to be seen, heard, and loved for who we truly are, not just the polished versions of ourselves we often present to the world.

In the following sections, we'll explore the importance of social connection, offer practical tips for building a supportive network, and guide you through an exercise that will help you reach out to someone you admire. Remember, connection is not a luxury; it's a necessity. It's time to prioritize those relationships that nourish your soul and support your journey to a more purposeful, regret-free life.

THE IMPORTANCE OF SOCIAL CONNECTION

Have you ever felt that warm glow after a heart-to-heart with a close friend, or the surge of joy when celebrating a milestone with loved ones? That's the power of social connection at work.

We humans are wired for connection. Think about it – from the moment we're born, we crave touch, eye contact, and interaction. As we grow, our need for meaningful relationships only deepens. We thrive in communities, families, and friendships, where we can share our joys, sorrows, and everything in between.

THE SCIENCE OF CONNECTION

Social connection isn't just a feel-good concept; it's essential for our health and well-being. Research has shown that strong social bonds are linked to a longer lifespan, lower rates of depression and anxiety, and a stronger immune system. When

we feel connected to others, our brains release oxytocin, a hormone that reduces stress and promotes feelings of trust and bonding.

On the flip side, loneliness and isolation can have devastating consequences. Research has linked social isolation to increased risk of heart disease, stroke, and even dementia. Feeling alone can also trigger negative thought patterns, exacerbate stress, and make challenges feel insurmountable.

YOUR SUPPORT SYSTEM

Think of your supportive relationships as a safety net – they catch you when you fall, lift you when you're down, and celebrate with you when you soar. They provide a sounding board for your ideas, a shoulder to cry on when things get tough, and a source of encouragement when you need it most.

Here are just a few ways supportive relationships can enrich your life:

- **Navigating Challenges:** When we face challenges, having someone to turn to can make all the difference. Whether it's a listening ear, a different perspective, or practical help, supportive relationships can help us find solutions and persevere.

- **Celebrating Successes:** Sharing our achievements with loved ones amplifies our joy and reinforces our sense of accomplishment. Supportive friends and family celebrate our wins with us, big and small, boosting our confidence and motivation.
- **Emotional Support:** A listening ear, a comforting hug, or a few words of encouragement can go a long way in helping us manage difficult emotions. Supportive relationships provide a safe space for us to express our feelings and receive empathy and understanding.
- **Personal Growth:** Our relationships challenge us to grow, learn, and evolve. They expose us to new ideas, perspectives, and ways of being, pushing us beyond our comfort zones and helping us become the best version of ourselves.
- **Sense of Belonging:** Feeling like we belong to a community or a group of friends gives us a sense of identity and purpose. It reminds us that we're not alone in this journey and that we have people who care about us and our well-being.

BUILDING YOUR CIRCLE OF SUPPORT

While some of us are fortunate to have strong social connections already in place, others may need to put in more effort to build their circle of support. Here are some tips:

- **Reach Out to Existing Connections:** Reconnect with

old friends, family members, or colleagues. Schedule regular coffee dates, phone calls, or video chats to stay in touch.
- **Join Social Groups or Clubs:** Find groups that align with your interests, hobbies, or values. This could be a book club, a sports team, a volunteer organization, or a faith-based community.
- **Be a Good Listener:** One of the best ways to build strong relationships is to be a good listener. Show genuine interest in others, ask thoughtful questions, and offer support and encouragement.
- **Give Back:** Volunteering or helping others is a great way to meet new people and build connections while making a positive impact on the world.
- **Be Open and Authentic:** Don't be afraid to show your true self. Share your thoughts, feelings, and experiences with others. Vulnerability fosters deeper connections.

Remember, building meaningful relationships takes time and effort. Don't get discouraged if you don't see results overnight. Just keep showing up, being yourself, and investing in the connections that matter most to you.

BUILDING A SUPPORTIVE NETWORK

Think of your support network as a sturdy bridge that helps you cross the turbulent waters of life. It's made up of the people who lift you up, believe in you, and encourage you to become the best version of yourself. These are the folks who cheer you on when you succeed, offer a shoulder to lean on when you're down, and provide a safe space for you to be your authentic self.

Having a strong support network is crucial for living a regret-free, purpose-driven life. When you're surrounded by people who genuinely care about you, you're more likely to take risks, pursue your dreams, and navigate life's challenges with resilience and grace. But how exactly do you build and nurture such a network? Let's dive into some practical tips:

1. **Reconnect with Loved Ones:** Sometimes, the strongest connections are the ones closest to home. Reach out to family members, old friends, or colleagues you've lost touch with. A simple phone call, a heartfelt letter, or a coffee date can rekindle those bonds and remind you of the love and support that's already in your life.
2. **Join Social Groups:** Look for groups or communities that align with your interests, hobbies, or values. This could be a book club, a sports team, a volunteer organization, a faith-based group, or even an online community. These shared experiences can create instant connections and foster meaningful relationships.
3. **Seek Out Mentors:** A mentor is someone who has achieved what you aspire to and who can offer guidance, advice, and support. They can share their wisdom, insights, and experiences, helping you navigate your own path with greater clarity and confidence. Look for mentors within your field, community, or personal network. Don't be afraid to ask for their guidance—most people are honored to be asked and happy to help.
4. **Be a Good Friend:** Building a strong support network

is a two-way street. Be the kind of friend you want to have. Show up for others, listen actively, offer help when needed, and celebrate their successes. Genuine connections are built on mutual respect, trust, and reciprocity.

5. **Set Boundaries:** Healthy relationships require healthy boundaries. It's okay to say no to requests that drain your energy or don't align with your values. It's also okay to distance yourself from people who are negative or toxic. Protect your energy and prioritize relationships that uplift and empower you.

6. **Be Open to New Connections:** Sometimes, the most unexpected people can become our greatest supporters. Be open to meeting new people and forming connections with those who are different from you. You never know who might inspire you, challenge you, or become a lifelong friend.

7. **Nurture Your Relationships:** Relationships, like plants, need care and attention to thrive. Make time for the people who matter to you. Schedule regular phone calls, coffee dates, or walks. Send thoughtful notes or messages. Celebrate milestones and special occasions together. The more you invest in your relationships, the stronger they will become.

8. **Communicate Openly and Honestly:** Strong relationships are built on a foundation of open communication. Share your thoughts, feelings, and experiences with your loved ones. Be willing to listen to their perspectives and offer support in return. Honest communication builds trust and deepens connection.

9. **Offer Support and Encouragement:** Be there for your loved ones when they need you. Offer a listening ear, a helping hand, or a shoulder to cry on. Celebrate their successes and encourage them to pursue their dreams. Remember, the support you give is just as important as the support you receive.
10. **Forgive and Let Go:** In any relationship, there will be times when you feel hurt, disappointed, or let down. Practice forgiveness, both for yourself and for others. Holding onto grudges only poisons your heart and damages your relationships. Let go of past hurts and focus on building a brighter future together.

Building a supportive network takes time and effort, but the rewards are immeasurable. Surround yourself with people who believe in you, uplift you, and inspire you to be your best self. These relationships will not only enrich your life but also empower you to live a life of purpose, passion, and no regrets.

EXERCISE: REACH OUT TO SOMEONE YOU ADMIRE

Who inspires you? Who do you look up to? Who has achieved something you aspire to?

This exercise is about connecting with that person. It's about reaching out to someone you admire, whether it's a friend, family member, colleague, or even a public figure you've never met. It's about opening the door to mentorship, guidance, and inspiration.

WHY REACH OUT?

Connecting with someone you admire can be incredibly beneficial. It can:

- **Provide valuable insights and advice:** This person has likely walked a path similar to the one you're on. They can offer you wisdom, guidance, and support based on their own experiences.
- **Expand your network:** Building relationships with inspiring individuals can open doors to new opportunities and collaborations.
- **Boost your confidence:** Hearing from someone you admire that they believe in you can give you a tremendous boost of confidence and motivation.
- **Inspire you to take action:** Seeing someone else achieve their dreams can ignite your own passion and drive.

HOW TO REACH OUT

Reaching out can feel intimidating, but it doesn't have to be. Here are a few simple steps:

1. **Identify who you admire:** Think about who inspires you and why. What qualities or achievements do they possess that you admire?
2. **Choose your method of contact:** Consider the best way to reach out. If it's someone you know personally, a phone call, email, or in-person meeting might be

appropriate. If it's someone you don't know, consider sending a thoughtful email or message on social media.
3. **Craft your message:** Keep it concise and focused. Briefly introduce yourself, express your admiration for their work or achievements, and explain why you're reaching out. If you're requesting a meeting or conversation, be specific about what you're hoping to learn or discuss.
4. **Be genuine and respectful:** Express your admiration authentically and respectfully. Remember, you're asking for their time and attention, so be polite and appreciative.
5. **Follow up:** If you don't hear back right away, don't be discouraged. Follow up once or twice, but be respectful of their time and don't be pushy.

WHAT TO SAY

Here are some examples of what you could say in your message:

- "Hi [Name], I've been following your work for a while now and I'm so inspired by your [achievement/quality]. I'd love to hear more about your journey and get your advice on [topic]."
- "Dear [Name], I'm a huge fan of your [book/podcast/project]. Your work has really resonated with me because [reason]. I'd be honored if you'd be willing to have a brief conversation with me about [topic]."
- "Hello [Name], I'm reaching out to you because I'm

looking for a mentor in [field]. Your experience and expertise in [area] are truly impressive. I'd love to learn from you and get your guidance on [topic]."

OVERCOMING HESITATION

If you're feeling hesitant about reaching out, here are a few tips to help you overcome your fear:

- **Remember, they were once in your shoes:** Everyone starts somewhere. The person you admire was once a beginner too. They may be more than willing to help you along your journey.
- **Think about what you have to offer:** Even if you're just starting out, you have unique experiences and perspectives to share. Don't underestimate the value of your own insights and questions.
- **Focus on the potential benefits:** The worst that can happen is that they say no. But the best that can happen is that you gain a mentor, valuable advice, and a new connection.
- **Be brave:** Taking the initiative to reach out shows confidence and drive. It's a step towards taking ownership of your own growth and development.

YOUR TURN

Now it's your turn to take action. Who do you admire? What do you want to learn from them? Don't let fear or hesitation hold you back. Reach out and see what happens.

You might be surprised at how willing people are to help and inspire.

Remember, living with intention means taking bold steps towards your goals and dreams. Reaching out to someone you admire is a powerful way to do just that. So, go ahead and send that email, make that phone call, or strike up a conversation. You have nothing to lose and everything to gain.

Day 27: Learn and Grow

Remember that feeling when you first learned to ride a bike, or maybe when you finally mastered that tricky guitar chord? That sense of accomplishment, of expanding your horizons and stepping into a new realm of possibility? That, my friend, is the magic of learning.

It's easy to fall into the trap of thinking that our formal education is the end of our learning journey. We graduate high school, college, maybe even get a few certifications under our belt, and then we think, "Okay, I'm done. I know enough."

But the truth is, our potential for growth and learning is limitless. And I'm not just talking about earning another degree or adding to your resume. I'm talking about the kind of learning that sparks curiosity, ignites passion, and expands your understanding of the world and yourself.

Learning isn't just about acquiring knowledge; it's about evolving into the best version of yourself. It's about challenging your assumptions, broadening your perspectives, and discovering hidden talents and passions you never knew you had.

When we commit to lifelong learning, we open ourselves

up to a world of possibilities. We become more adaptable, resilient, and creative. We discover new ways to contribute to the world and make a positive impact. We also keep our minds sharp, our spirits vibrant, and our lives filled with purpose and meaning.

Think of it like this: your mind is a muscle. The more you use it, the stronger it gets. And just like physical exercise keeps your body healthy, mental exercise keeps your mind agile and adaptable.

The beauty of learning is that it can take many forms. It can be as simple as reading a book, listening to a podcast, or having a conversation with someone who has a different perspective. It can involve taking a course, learning a new skill, or exploring a new hobby.

No matter how you choose to learn, the most important thing is to make it a priority. Carve out time in your schedule for learning, just like you would for exercise or spending time with loved ones. Invest in yourself and your growth.

Remember, learning is not just about what you know; it's about who you become. It's about expanding your horizons, challenging your limits, and discovering the full potential of your mind and spirit.

So let's dive into the world of lifelong learning and explore how it can transform your life and empower you to live with purpose and passion.

THE VALUE OF LIFELONG LEARNING

Remember that feeling of excitement when you learned something new as a child? Maybe it was the thrill of riding a bike without training wheels, the satisfaction of reading your first chapter book, or the pride of solving a complex math problem. Learning was an adventure, a journey of discovery that expanded your world and ignited your curiosity.

But somewhere along the way, for many of us, that spark began to fade. We started to associate learning with school, tests, and pressure. We convinced ourselves that once we graduated, our learning days were behind us.

What a tragedy!

Because here's the truth: learning isn't just for kids. It's a lifelong pursuit, a continuous journey that enriches our lives, expands our minds, and keeps us vibrant and engaged. Lifelong learning isn't about earning degrees or accumulating knowledge for the sake of it; it's about personal growth, self-discovery, and unlocking our full potential.

THE BENEFITS OF LIFELONG LEARNING

So, why should we make lifelong learning a priority? Let me share a few compelling reasons:

1. **Boosts Brainpower:** Learning new things creates new neural pathways in our brains, keeping them active and healthy. It's like exercise for our minds, helping us stay sharp, focused, and mentally agile as we age.
2. **Ignites Curiosity:** When we learn, we open ourselves up to new ideas, perspectives, and possibilities. We cultivate a sense of wonder and curiosity that keeps us engaged with the world around us.
3. **Enhances Adaptability:** In today's fast-paced, ever-

changing world, adaptability is key. Lifelong learning helps us develop the skills and mindset needed to navigate change, embrace new challenges, and thrive in any environment.

4. **Fosters Confidence:** Acquiring new knowledge and skills builds self-efficacy, the belief in our ability to succeed. This increased confidence can empower us to take on new challenges, pursue our goals, and step outside our comfort zones.
5. **Enriches Life:** Learning new things simply makes life more interesting and fulfilling. Whether it's picking up a new hobby, exploring a different culture, or mastering a new skill, continuous learning adds depth and richness to our experiences.
6. **Expands Career Opportunities:** In today's competitive job market, the ability to learn new skills quickly is a valuable asset. Lifelong learners are more likely to be sought after by employers, as they are adaptable, versatile, and always willing to grow.

HOW TO EMBRACE LIFELONG LEARNING

Now that we've established the "why," let's talk about the "how." How can you make lifelong learning a part of your daily life?

1. **Cultivate Curiosity:** Be open to new ideas and perspectives. Ask questions, explore different viewpoints, and challenge your assumptions.
2. **Set Learning Goals:** What do you want to learn? It

could be anything from a new language to a musical instrument to a business skill. Set specific, measurable goals to keep yourself motivated and on track.

3. **Explore Your Interests:** What are you passionate about? What sparks your curiosity? Dive into those interests. Take a class, read books, watch documentaries, or find a mentor who can share their knowledge and expertise.
4. **Make it a Habit:** Set aside time each day or week for learning. This could involve reading for 30 minutes, listening to a podcast during your commute, or taking an online course.
5. **Be Resourceful:** There are countless resources available for learning, many of them free or low-cost. Take advantage of online courses, libraries, workshops, webinars, and educational apps.
6. **Embrace Technology:** Technology has revolutionized the way we learn. Use online platforms, social media, and educational apps to connect with experts, discover new resources, and learn at your own pace.
7. **Find a Learning Community:** Connect with others who share your passion for learning. Join book clubs, discussion groups, or online communities where you can exchange ideas, share resources, and support each other's learning journeys.
8. **Celebrate Your Progress:** Acknowledge your achievements, no matter how small. Each step you take on your learning journey is a victory worth celebrating.

BREAKING DOWN BARRIERS TO LEARNING

It's important to acknowledge that there may be obstacles that get in the way of lifelong learning. Perhaps you feel like you don't have enough time, money, or energy. Maybe you're worried about failing or looking foolish. Or perhaps you simply don't know where to start.

Remember, everyone faces challenges. But these obstacles don't have to hold you back. With a little creativity and determination, you can find ways to overcome them. If time is an issue, try incorporating learning into your daily routine. Listen to educational podcasts while you commute, read during your lunch break, or take online courses in the evenings.

If money is a concern, there are plenty of free or low-cost learning resources available. Libraries, online courses, and community centers often offer workshops and classes at affordable prices. You can also find a wealth of information online through blogs, podcasts, and YouTube videos.

And if you're afraid of failure or looking foolish, remember that everyone starts somewhere. Don't be afraid to ask for help, seek out mentors, and embrace the learning process as an adventure.

CONCLUSION

Lifelong learning is not a luxury; it's a necessity for personal growth, fulfillment, and success in today's world. It's a journey of self-discovery, a way to expand our horizons, challenge our assumptions, and become the best versions of ourselves.

LEARNING FOR PURPOSE

Remember that spark of excitement you felt when you first discovered your purpose? That feeling of possibility, of knowing you're on the right path? Learning is the fuel that keeps that spark alive.

Think of your purpose as a garden. You've planted the seeds of your dreams, and now it's time to nurture them. Learning is the sunshine and water that nourishes those seeds, helping them grow into strong, vibrant plants.

But here's the thing: learning isn't just about acquiring knowledge for the sake of it. It's about seeking out opportunities that align with your passions and goals. It's about fueling your purpose with the information, skills, and insights that will help you thrive.

WHY LEARNING MATTERS FOR YOUR PURPOSE

1. **Stay Relevant and Adaptable:** The world is constantly changing, and so are the needs and challenges associated with your purpose. By continuously learning, you stay ahead of the curve, adapt to new trends, and remain relevant in your field.
2. **Expand Your Skill Set:** New skills open up new possibilities. Whether it's mastering a new software program, learning a foreign language, or honing your communication skills, each new skill expands your toolkit for living your purpose.
3. **Boost Your Confidence:** Learning something new is

empowering. It reminds you that you're capable of growth and challenges you to step outside your comfort zone. This increased confidence spills over into other areas of your life, fueling your pursuit of purpose.

4. **Connect with Like-Minded People:** Learning environments provide opportunities to connect with others who share your passions and interests. These connections can lead to valuable collaborations, mentorship opportunities, and a sense of community.
5. **Fuel Your Creativity:** Learning sparks new ideas and fresh perspectives. It helps you think outside the box, solve problems creatively, and approach your purpose with renewed enthusiasm.

DESIGNING YOUR LEARNING JOURNEY

Your learning journey is unique to you. There's no one-size-fits-all approach. The key is to be intentional and strategic about how you invest your time and energy.

Here are some practical ways to seek out learning opportunities that align with your purpose:

- **Take a Course:** Online or in-person courses are a great way to delve deep into a specific topic and gain structured knowledge. Look for courses that directly relate to your purpose or that teach you new skills that can enhance your work.
- **Read Books:** Books are a treasure trove of wisdom and inspiration. Choose books that challenge you to think

differently, expand your knowledge base, or provide practical guidance on living a purposeful life.
- **Attend Workshops or Conferences:** These events offer opportunities to learn from experts in your field, network with like-minded people, and gain fresh insights that can fuel your purpose.
- **Find a Mentor:** A mentor can provide valuable guidance, support, and encouragement as you navigate your purpose journey. Seek out someone you admire who has achieved success in a field related to yours.
- **Join Online Communities:** Connect with others who share your passions through online forums, Facebook groups, or LinkedIn groups. These communities can be a great source of information, support, and inspiration.
- **Listen to Podcasts or Webinars:** Podcasts and webinars are convenient ways to learn on the go. Look for shows or presentations that offer insights into your field, personal development, or living a purposeful life.
- **Volunteer or Intern:** Hands-on experience can be an incredibly valuable learning opportunity. Volunteering or interning in a field related to your purpose allows you to gain practical skills, make connections, and test the waters before fully diving in.

Remember, learning doesn't have to be formal or expensive. It can be as simple as reading an article online, listening to a TED Talk, or having a conversation with someone knowledgeable in your field. The key is to be curious, open-minded, and actively seek out opportunities to expand your knowledge and skills.

EMBRACE THE GROWTH MINDSET

The most important ingredient in your learning journey is a growth mindset. This means believing that your abilities and intelligence can be developed through dedication and hard work. People with a growth mindset embrace challenges, persist in the face of setbacks, and see effort as a path to mastery.

When you approach learning with a growth mindset, you view mistakes as opportunities for learning, not as signs of failure. You seek out feedback and use it to improve. You're not afraid to ask for help when you need it.

MAKE LEARNING A LIFELONG HABIT

Learning shouldn't stop after this 30-day challenge. Make it a lifelong commitment. Carve out time in your schedule for regular learning activities. Set learning goals and track your progress. Celebrate your achievements and reflect on the lessons you've learned.

Remember, the more you learn, the more you grow. And the more you grow, the closer you'll get to living a life that is truly aligned with your purpose.

EXERCISE: LEARNING PLAN

Welcome to the exciting part – creating your personal roadmap for growth and learning! Remember, living a purposeful life involves continuous evolution, and there's no better way to do that than by expanding your knowledge and skills. So, let's dive in and design a learning plan that will ignite your curiosity and propel you towards your dreams.

WHY CREATE A LEARNING PLAN?

Think of your learning plan as a compass guiding you towards a more fulfilling and purposeful life. By setting clear learning goals and outlining specific actions, you're not just wandering aimlessly; you're charting a deliberate course for your personal and professional development.

A well-crafted learning plan can:

- **Boost your confidence:** Mastering new skills empowers you and reinforces your belief in your abilities.
- **Open up new opportunities:** Learning expands your horizons, exposing you to possibilities you might not have considered before.
- **Enhance your problem-solving skills:** Knowledge equips you with different perspectives and approaches to tackle challenges.
- **Keep you engaged and motivated:** Learning something new is inherently exciting and can reignite your passion for life.

Step 1: Identify Your Learning Goals Take a moment to reflect on your passions, interests, and areas where you'd like to grow. What skills or knowledge would enhance your life, career, or personal development? What topics spark your curiosity and make you want to learn more?

Don't feel pressured to choose something purely practical

or career-oriented. This is your personal learning journey, so feel free to explore whatever excites you. Maybe you've always wanted to learn a new language, master a musical instrument, delve into the world of art, or understand the intricacies of coding. The possibilities are endless!

Choose 1-2 specific learning goals that resonate with you. Remember, it's better to focus on a few key areas and master them than to spread yourself too thin across multiple disciplines.

Step 2: Create a SMART Action Plan Now that you have your learning goals in mind, it's time to create a concrete plan for achieving them. Remember those SMART goals we talked about earlier? Let's apply that framework here:

- **Specific:** Clearly define what you want to learn. Instead of saying, "I want to learn about photography," be specific: "I want to learn how to take professional-quality portraits using natural light."
- **Measurable:** Set clear milestones or benchmarks to track your progress. For example, "I will complete an online photography course with a passing grade within one month."
- **Achievable:** Be realistic about what you can accomplish in the given timeframe. Start small and build upon your successes.
- **Relevant:** Ensure your learning goals align with your overall purpose and values. How will this new knowledge or skill contribute to your personal growth or professional development?
- **Time-Bound:** Set a deadline for achieving your goals.

This creates a sense of urgency and helps you stay focused.

Step 3: Gather Your Resources Now that you have a clear plan, it's time to gather the resources you'll need to support your learning journey. Depending on your chosen skills or knowledge areas, your resources might include:

- **Books:** Explore libraries, bookstores, or online retailers for books on your topic of interest.
- **Online courses:** Platforms like Coursera, Udemy, Skillshare, and LinkedIn Learning offer a vast array of courses on virtually any subject.
- **Mentors or coaches:** Seek out experts in your field who can offer guidance, advice, and support.
- **Workshops or conferences:** Attend events where you can learn from experts and network with like-minded individuals.
- **Online communities:** Join forums or social media groups dedicated to your chosen subject to connect with others who share your passion.

Step 4: Schedule Dedicated Learning Time Treat your learning journey like any other important commitment. Block out specific times in your schedule dedicated to learning. Even 30 minutes a day can make a significant difference over time. Experiment with different times of day to find what works best for you. Some people prefer to learn in the morning when their minds are fresh, while others find evenings more conducive to focus.

Step 5: Track Your Progress and Celebrate Wins Keep track of your learning progress using a journal, spreadsheet, or app. Note down your accomplishments, challenges, and any new insights or ideas that arise. Celebrate your milestones along the way. Acknowledging your progress reinforces positive behavior and keeps you motivated.

Step 6: Adapt and Evolve Remember, your learning plan is not set in stone. It's a dynamic tool that you can adjust and refine as you go. Be flexible and open to adapting your plan based on your experience, interests, and changing circumstances. Don't be afraid to experiment with different learning styles or resources. The key is to find what works best for you and enjoy the process of learning and growing.

So, there you have it – your personalized learning plan. Embrace it, commit to it, and watch as you unlock your full potential, one step at a time. Remember, learning is not just about acquiring knowledge; it's about transforming yourself and creating a life filled with purpose, passion, and endless possibilities.

Day 28: Embrace Change

Buckle up, friend, because today we're tackling a big one: change.

Change is inevitable. It's the only constant in life, as the saying goes. It can be as subtle as the seasons shifting or as dramatic as a sudden life event. It can bring excitement and opportunity, or it can bring uncertainty and fear.

But here's the thing: resisting change is like trying to hold back the tide. It's exhausting, futile, and ultimately keeps us stuck. Embracing change, on the other hand, is like riding a wave. It's exhilarating, empowering, and opens up a world of possibilities.

Think back to a time in your life when you experienced a significant change. Maybe it was a new job, a move to a new city, the end of a relationship, or a personal transformation. It probably wasn't easy, but you got through it. You adapted, you learned, you grew.

That resilience you showed is your superpower. It's the ability to bend without breaking, to find your footing in shifting sands, and to emerge stronger from adversity. It's the key to living a regret-free life.

THE RESISTANCE TO CHANGE

Why do we resist change so fiercely? It often boils down to fear. Fear of the unknown, fear of failure, fear of losing control. We cling to the familiar because it feels safe, even if it's no longer serving us.

But here's the paradox: the things we fear the most are often the very things we need to grow. Change forces us to step outside our comfort zones, to confront our limitations, and to discover new strengths within ourselves.

Resisting change not only holds us back from personal growth; it also keeps us stuck in the past. We replay old regrets, cling to outdated beliefs, and miss out on new opportunities.

THE POWER OF EMBRACING CHANGE

Embracing change doesn't mean you have to love every unexpected turn life throws your way. It simply means accepting that change is a part of life and choosing to adapt rather than resist.

When we embrace change, we open ourselves up to new experiences, perspectives, and possibilities. We learn to trust our ability to navigate the unknown, to bounce back from setbacks, and to create a life that is constantly evolving and expanding.

Embracing change also means letting go of the need for control. It means surrendering to the flow of life, trusting that even the most challenging experiences can lead to growth and transformation.

In today's exercise, we'll explore how to embrace change as a catalyst for growth. You'll learn to reframe your perspective, shift your mindset, and develop strategies for navigating life's transitions with grace and resilience. Get ready to step out of your comfort zone and into a world of endless possibilities!

THE INEVITABILITY OF CHANGE

Picture this: You're standing on the shore, watching the waves roll in and out, each one different from the last. The tide rises and falls, the sun moves across the sky, and the weather shifts from sunny to stormy and back again. This is the rhythm of nature, the constant ebb and flow of change.

Just like the ocean, our lives are in a state of perpetual motion. We grow, we learn, we evolve. Our circumstances shift, our relationships change, and our priorities evolve. Change is not an anomaly; it's the very fabric of our existence.

Yet, despite the inevitability of change, we often resist it with all our might. We cling to the familiar, crave stability, and fear the unknown. We build walls around our comfort zones, hoping to shield ourselves from the winds of change. But here's the truth: resisting change is like trying to stop the tide with a sandcastle. It's a futile effort that only leads to frustration, stress, and unhappiness.

Think about a time in your life when you resisted change. Perhaps it was a job loss, a breakup, or a move to a new city. How did that resistance feel? Did it make the situation easier or more difficult? Did it open up new possibilities or keep you stuck in the past?

When we resist change, we create unnecessary suffering. We fight against the natural flow of life, exhausting ourselves in the process. We miss out on opportunities for growth, new experiences, and a deeper understanding of ourselves.

EMBRACING CHANGE: A PATH TO GROWTH AND OPPORTUNITY

What if, instead of resisting change, we embraced it? What if we saw it as a natural part of life, a chance to learn, grow, and evolve? What if we opened our hearts and minds to the possibilities that change brings?

Embracing change doesn't mean that we have to like or agree with every shift that comes our way. It simply means that we accept it as a reality, that we acknowledge it as a part of life's journey.

When we embrace change, we open ourselves up to a world of opportunities. We allow ourselves to step outside of our comfort zones, try new things, and discover hidden talents. We become more resilient, adaptable, and creative.

Think of the butterfly. It starts as a caterpillar, confined to its cocoon. But through the process of metamorphosis, it transforms into a beautiful creature capable of flight. This transformation is only possible because the caterpillar embraces change.

Change can be scary, but it's also exciting. It forces us to re-evaluate our priorities, redefine our goals, and discover new paths. It pushes us to become the best version of ourselves.

HOW TO EMBRACE CHANGE:

Embracing change is a process that requires courage, openness, and a willingness to let go of the past. Here are a few tips to help you navigate the winds of change with grace and resilience:

1. **Acknowledge Your Feelings:** It's okay to feel scared, sad, or angry when faced with change. Allow yourself to feel those emotions fully, without judgment.
2. **Challenge Your Assumptions:** Question your beliefs about change. Are they based on fear or reality? Are there other ways to view the situation?
3. **Focus on What You Can Control:** You may not be able to control the external circumstances, but you can control your attitude and response. Choose to focus on the positive aspects of change and the opportunities it presents.
4. **Seek Support:** Don't go through it alone. Reach out to loved ones, friends, or a therapist for support and guidance.
5. **Practice Self-Care:** Take care of your physical, emotional, and mental well-being during times of change. Eat healthy, exercise, get enough sleep, and engage in activities that bring you joy.
6. **Celebrate Small Wins:** Acknowledge and celebrate every small victory along the way. This will help you stay motivated and positive as you navigate the transition.

Remember, change is not a sign of weakness or failure. It's

a sign that you're alive, that you're growing, and that you're capable of incredible transformation. By embracing change, you open yourself up to a world of possibilities and create a life that is rich, meaningful, and full of purpose.

NAVIGATING TRANSITIONS

Life is a series of transitions, both big and small. Some transitions are exciting, like starting a new job or moving to a new city. Others are challenging, like ending a relationship or dealing with a health issue. No matter what kind of transition you're facing, it's important to have strategies in place to navigate the ups and downs.

Think of transitions as a bridge between where you've been and where you're going. Like any bridge, there are bumps, curves, and perhaps even a few detours. But with the right tools and mindset, you can cross that bridge with confidence and arrive on the other side stronger and more resilient than ever before.

SETTING NEW GOALS: YOUR COMPASS FOR CHANGE

One of the most powerful strategies for navigating transitions is to set new goals. Goals give you a sense of direction and purpose, helping you stay focused and motivated during times of change. They provide a roadmap for where you want to go and what you want to achieve.

When setting new goals during a transition, it's important to be realistic and flexible. Don't put too much pressure on yourself to achieve everything at once. Start with small, achievable goals that will build your confidence and momentum.

Your goals should also be aligned with your values and purpose. What matters most to you? What kind of impact do you want to make in the world? When your goals are rooted in your deeper values, they become more meaningful and motivating.

SEEKING SUPPORT FROM LOVED ONES: YOUR LIFELINE

Transitions can be isolating, but you don't have to go through them alone. Reach out to your loved ones for support. Talk to your partner, friends, family, or a trusted mentor. Share your fears, anxieties, and hopes. Sometimes, just talking about what you're going through can make a world of difference.

Your loved ones can offer a listening ear, a shoulder to cry on, or practical advice and assistance. They can remind you of your strengths, offer words of encouragement, and help you stay grounded during challenging times.

Remember, asking for help is not a sign of weakness. It's a sign of strength and courage. It takes vulnerability to admit that you need support, but it's a crucial step towards navigating transitions successfully.

PRACTICING SELF-CARE: YOUR FOUNDATION FOR WELL-BEING

During times of change, it's essential to prioritize your

self-care. When we're stressed or overwhelmed, it's easy to neglect our own needs. But taking care of yourself physically, mentally, and emotionally is crucial for staying resilient and navigating transitions with grace.

Make time for activities that nourish your soul. Spend time in nature, read a good book, listen to music you love, or pursue a hobby. Take care of your body by eating nourishing foods, exercising regularly, and getting enough sleep. And don't forget to nurture your mind by practicing mindfulness, journaling, or engaging in other activities that promote mental well-being.

Remember, self-care is not selfish. It's essential for maintaining your energy, focus, and resilience. When you take care of yourself, you're better equipped to handle challenges, make sound decisions, and navigate through transitions with clarity and confidence.

EMBRACING THE JOURNEY

Transitions are an inevitable part of life. They can be challenging, but they also offer opportunities for growth, transformation, and new beginnings. By setting new goals, seeking support from loved ones, and practicing self-care, you can navigate transitions with greater ease and emerge on the other side stronger, wiser, and more aligned with your purpose.

Remember, the journey is just as important as the destination. Embrace the ups and downs, learn from your experiences, and trust that you have the strength and resilience to navigate any transition that comes your way.

By following these strategies and making self-care a

priority, you'll not only survive transitions but thrive through them. So embrace the journey, my friend, and let the winds of change carry you towards a brighter future.

EXERCISE: CHANGE REFLECTION

Change is an inevitable part of life. It's the one constant we can always count on, whether we like it or not. Sometimes change is welcome, bringing with it new opportunities and excitement. Other times, change can feel overwhelming, scary, or even devastating.

Think back to a time in your life when you experienced a significant change. It could be a career change, a move to a new city, the end of a relationship, the birth of a child, or any other event that shifted the landscape of your life.

Remember how it felt in the beginning. Did you feel excited? Scared? Confused? Overwhelmed? Maybe a mix of all of the above? Change, even positive change, can often trigger a range of emotions.

Now, I want you to take a few moments to reflect on how you navigated that change. What strategies did you use to cope? What mindset shifts helped you adapt and move forward? How did you overcome any challenges or setbacks that arose along the way?

Perhaps you found solace in talking to a trusted friend or family member. Maybe you sought professional guidance from a therapist or coach. Perhaps you immersed yourself in a new hobby or activity to distract yourself from the stress of the transition. Or maybe you simply took things one day at a time, focusing on putting one foot in front of the other.

Whatever your strategies, they worked! You successfully navigated that change, and you emerged on the other side stronger, wiser, and more resilient. That experience is a valuable asset, a testament to your ability to adapt and overcome adversity.

Now, let's dig a little deeper. I want you to consider the following questions:

1. What were the key mindset shifts that helped you through that change? Did you adopt a more positive outlook? Did you learn to let go of control? Did you embrace uncertainty?
2. What specific actions or behaviors did you take to manage the transition? Did you create a plan? Did you set small, achievable goals? Did you seek support from others?
3. What lessons did you learn from that experience? Did you discover hidden strengths or resources within yourself? Did you gain a new perspective on life?
4. How can you apply those lessons to future changes? What strategies or mindset shifts can you carry with you to navigate upcoming transitions with more ease and confidence?

Take some time to journal about your answers to these questions. Be as specific and detailed as possible. The more you understand your past experiences with change, the better equipped you'll be to face future changes with courage and optimism.

Remember, change is not something to be feared, but

rather an opportunity for growth and transformation. By reflecting on your past experiences with change, you can identify the tools and resources you already possess to successfully navigate any transition that comes your way.

Here are some additional prompts to guide your reflection:

- What were the most challenging aspects of that change?
- How did you overcome those challenges?
- What were the most positive aspects of that change?
- How did you embrace those positive aspects?
- What advice would you give to someone going through a similar change?

By taking the time to reflect on your past experiences with change, you're not only honoring your resilience and growth, but you're also creating a roadmap for the future. You're reminding yourself that you have the inner strength and wisdom to navigate any transition that life throws your way. And that, my friend, is a truly empowering realization.

As you continue on your journey of purposeful living, remember that change is a constant companion. But armed with self-awareness, resilience, and the right tools, you can embrace change as an opportunity to evolve, learn, and grow.

Day 29: Trust Your Intuition

Have you ever had a gut feeling about something, a hunch that turned out to be right? Or perhaps you've ignored that inner voice only to regret it later? That's your intuition speaking, a powerful internal compass that can guide you towards your true path and help you make decisions that align with your deepest values and desires.

Intuition, often described as a "gut feeling" or a "knowing," is that subtle whisper within that goes beyond logic and reason. It's a wisdom that comes from deep within, a synthesis of our experiences, emotions, and instincts. Yet, in a world that often values intellect and analysis, it's easy to dismiss or ignore our intuitive insights.

Today, we're going to dive into the power of intuition and learn how to tap into this invaluable resource. We'll explore what intuition is, how it manifests in our lives, and why it's so important to trust it, especially as we navigate our purpose-driven journey.

Why Intuition Matters

Think of your intuition as your internal GPS system.

It's constantly receiving signals and information from your environment, your subconscious mind, and even your body. These signals, often subtle and fleeting, can provide valuable insights and guidance when we're faced with decisions or challenges.

Trusting your intuition doesn't mean abandoning logic or reason. It's about finding a balance between the head and the heart, between analysis and instinct. When we learn to listen to our intuition, we gain access to a deeper level of wisdom and understanding that can guide us towards the choices that are truly right for us.

THE BENEFITS OF TRUSTING YOUR INTUITION

- **Enhanced Decision-Making:** Intuition can help us make decisions quickly and confidently, even when faced with limited information or complex situations.
- **Increased Self-Trust:** When we honor our intuition, we build trust in ourselves and our ability to make sound judgments.
- **Improved Well-being:** Tuning into our intuition can reduce stress, anxiety, and overwhelm by guiding us towards choices that align with our values and needs.
- **Deeper Self-Awareness:** Intuition helps us connect with our authentic selves, understand our emotions, and make choices that honor our true desires.
- **Greater Authenticity:** By trusting our intuition, we're more likely to live a life that feels true to who we are, leading to greater fulfillment and happiness.

THE CHALLENGE OF TRUSTING INTUITION

Despite its many benefits, trusting our intuition can be a challenge. We may have been conditioned to doubt our gut feelings or to prioritize logic over instinct. Fear, self-doubt, and societal expectations can all cloud our ability to hear our inner voice.

But just like any skill, trusting your intuition takes practice. The more we tune in and honor our intuitive insights, the stronger and clearer they become. Over time, we can develop a deep trust in this inner wisdom that can guide us through life's challenges and lead us towards a more fulfilling and purposeful existence.

In this chapter, we'll explore practical techniques for cultivating and strengthening your intuition. You'll learn how to quiet the noise of the external world, listen to the subtle whispers of your inner voice, and make choices that align with your true self.

THE WISDOM WITHIN

Have you ever had a gut feeling about something? That nagging sense that you should or shouldn't do something, even if you couldn't quite explain why? That, my friend, is your intuition speaking to you.

Intuition is often described as our "inner knowing" or "gut feeling." It's a subtle, often unconscious wisdom that arises from deep within us, offering guidance and insights that go beyond logic and reason. Some call it a hunch, others a whisper from the soul. Whatever you call it, intuition is a powerful tool that can help you make decisions, navigate challenges, and live a more authentic and purposeful life.

Think of your intuition as a compass guiding you towards your true north. It's a wise, inner voice that knows what's best for you, even when your conscious mind is clouded with doubt or uncertainty. When you learn to tap into your intuition, you gain access to a wealth of wisdom and guidance that can lead you down the path of your highest potential.

But what exactly is intuition, and how does it work? While science is still unraveling the mysteries of intuition, researchers believe it's a complex process that involves both conscious and unconscious factors. Your intuition draws upon your past experiences, knowledge, emotions, and even your physical sensations to provide you with insights and guidance.

Think of it like this: your brain is constantly processing information, even when you're not consciously aware of it. Your intuition is like a filter that sifts through this vast amount of data, picking up on subtle patterns and connections that your conscious mind might miss. It then presents you with a "gut feeling" or a "knowing" that can guide your decisions and actions.

Why should you trust your intuition? Because it's often more accurate than you think. Studies have shown that people who trust their intuition tend to make better decisions, experience less stress, and have greater overall well-being.

Your intuition is not infallible, of course. It's important to use discernment and consider all available information before making any major decisions. But when you learn to listen to your intuition and trust its guidance, you'll be amazed at how often it leads you in the right direction.

HOW INTUITION GUIDES YOU TOWARDS YOUR PURPOSE

Your intuition is especially powerful when it comes to living a purposeful life. It's like having a built-in GPS system that knows the exact coordinates of your dreams and desires. When you're in tune with your intuition, you're more likely to make choices that align with your values, passions, and goals.

Have you ever felt a strong pull towards a certain career path or creative project, even if it seemed illogical or impractical? That's your intuition nudging you towards your purpose. It knows what will bring you the most fulfillment and satisfaction, even if it doesn't make sense on paper.

Your intuition can also help you navigate challenges and setbacks on your path to purpose. When you're faced with a difficult decision or a roadblock, your intuition can offer valuable insights and guidance. It can help you see the bigger picture, identify hidden opportunities, and make choices that are in your best interest.

For example, you might be considering a new job opportunity that looks good on paper but doesn't feel quite right. Your intuition might be telling you that the company culture isn't a good fit, or that the role wouldn't align with your values. By listening to this inner wisdom, you can avoid making a decision that you might later regret.

Similarly, your intuition can help you identify toxic relationships or situations that are no longer serving you. You might feel a sense of unease or discomfort around certain people or environments. Trusting these feelings can help you distance yourself from negativity and create space for more positive and supportive connections.

Learning to trust your intuition is like building a muscle. The more you use it, the stronger it becomes.

In the next section, we'll explore practical tips and exercises for strengthening your intuition and learning to trust its guidance.

HONORING YOUR INNER VOICE

Think back to a time you had a gut feeling about something. Maybe it was a job offer that looked great on paper, but something in your gut told you it wasn't right. Or perhaps it was a decision in your personal life where you felt a deep knowing, a sense of clarity that guided your choice. That, my friend, was your intuition speaking – your inner voice, your internal compass.

Our intuition is often described as a gut feeling, a hunch, or a knowing without conscious reasoning. It's a subtle whisper from our subconscious mind, drawing on our experiences, wisdom, and innate knowing. Yet, in a world that often prioritizes logic and reason, it's easy to dismiss our intuition as mere whimsy. But honoring our inner voice is a crucial step in living with intention and creating a life that truly aligns with our authentic selves.

So, how do we tune in to this inner compass? Here are some practical ways to cultivate and strengthen your intuition:

1. Practice Mindfulness: Mindfulness is the practice of being fully present in the moment, without judgment. It involves paying attention to our thoughts, feelings, and bodily sensations. When we're mindful, we create space for our intuition to emerge. We become more attuned to subtle signals from our bodies and emotions, which can often be masked by the noise of our busy minds.

Incorporating mindfulness into your daily routine can be as simple as taking a few deep breaths, focusing on your senses, or engaging in a meditation practice. By slowing down and tuning in, you'll start to notice the whispers of your intuition more clearly.

2. Listen to Your Body: Our bodies are incredibly wise. They often give us signals about what feels right and what doesn't. Have you ever felt a knot in your stomach before making a decision? Or a sense of lightness and ease when you're on the right path? These are your body's way of communicating with you.

Start paying attention to your physical sensations. Notice how your body reacts in different situations. Does your heart race when you're anxious? Do you feel a sense of warmth and expansion when you're excited? Learning to interpret your body's signals can provide valuable insights and guide you towards choices that resonate with your deepest needs and desires.

3. Pay Attention to Your Dreams: Dreams are often seen as a window into our subconscious mind. They can offer symbolic messages, creative solutions, and even warnings about potential pitfalls. Keeping a dream journal can help you decode the symbolism of your dreams and tap into their wisdom.

As you start paying attention to your dreams, you may notice recurring themes or images. These can provide valuable clues about your underlying emotions, desires, and fears. By exploring your dreams with curiosity and an open mind, you can unlock hidden insights and strengthen your intuition.

4. Trust Your Gut Feeling: When you feel a strong gut feeling about something, don't dismiss it. Take a moment to pause, reflect, and ask yourself, "What is my intuition trying to tell me?" Even if you can't logically explain it, trust that your gut feeling is based on a deeper wisdom.

Remember, your intuition is not always about predicting the future or making the "right" decision. It's about guiding you towards choices that are in alignment with your values, your authentic self, and your highest good.

5. Create Space for Silence: In our fast-paced, technology-driven world, it's easy to become overwhelmed by information and external stimuli. This constant bombardment can drown out our inner voice. Make time each day to disconnect from the noise and create space for silence.

This could involve spending time in nature, practicing meditation, or simply sitting quietly and allowing your thoughts to settle. By creating space for silence, you allow your intuition to surface and guide you.

6. Practice Intuitive Decision-Making: The more you practice listening to your intuition, the stronger it becomes. Start by making small decisions based on your gut feeling. Notice how it feels when you follow your intuition versus when you ignore it.

As you gain confidence in your intuition, you can start applying it to bigger decisions. Trust that your inner wisdom will guide you towards the path that is right for you.

THE GIFT OF INTUITION

Honoring your inner voice is a gift you give yourself. It's a way of saying, "I trust myself. I value my own wisdom and experience." When you honor your intuition, you become more aligned with your authentic self and make choices that lead to greater fulfillment and happiness.

It's important to remember that intuition is not a substitute for logic or reason. It's a complementary tool that can help us make more informed and aligned decisions. When we combine our intuition with our intellect, we create a powerful force for creating the life we desire.

EXERCISE: INTUITION CHECK-IN

In the whirlwind of daily life, it's easy to lose touch with our intuition – that quiet, inner voice that whispers wisdom and guidance. Yet, deep within each of us lies an innate knowing, a compass that can steer us towards decisions and actions that align with our truest selves. It's time to tune in and reconnect with your inner guide through this simple Intuition Check-In exercise.

Step 1: Create a Calm Space Find a quiet, comfortable space where you won't be disturbed. Turn off your phone, dim the lights, and create an atmosphere of tranquility. You might choose to light a candle, play soft music, or simply sit in silence.

Step 2: Relax Your Body Close your eyes and take a few deep breaths. Inhale slowly and deeply through your nose, filling your belly with air. Exhale slowly through your mouth, releasing any tension or stress. Feel your body relaxing with each breath.

Step 3: Focus on Your Question Bring to mind a current decision you're facing or a challenge you're experiencing. It could be a simple choice like where to go for dinner or a more complex issue like a career change or relationship concern. Clearly articulate your question in your mind.

Step 4: Tune into Your Body Pay attention to your body's sensations. Do you feel any tightness, tingling, or warmth anywhere? Does your gut feel relaxed or clenched? Do you have any intuitive "gut feelings" about the situation? Notice any subtle cues your body is sending you.

Step 5: Listen to Your Inner Voice Now, turn your attention inward and listen for your intuition's whisper. It may come as a fleeting thought, a knowingness, an image, or even a physical sensation. Don't try to force an answer; simply observe whatever arises in your mind and body.

Step 6: Journal Your Insights Open your eyes and take a few moments to jot down any insights, feelings, or sensations that came up during your check-in. Don't worry about analyzing or judging them; simply record them as they are.

ADDITIONAL TIPS FOR TUNING IN

- **Trust Your Gut:** Your intuition often communicates through your gut feelings. Pay attention to those sensations in your stomach, even if they don't make logical sense.
- **Notice Your Emotions:** Emotions can be valuable messengers of intuition. If you feel a sense of peace,

excitement, or alignment with a certain choice, that may be a sign that you're on the right track. Conversely, feelings of unease or disquiet could be a warning sign.
- **Be Patient:** Intuition doesn't always speak loudly or clearly. Sometimes it whispers, and sometimes it takes time for the message to become clear. Be patient with yourself and trust the process.
- **Practice Regularly:** The more you practice tuning into your intuition, the stronger and clearer it will become. Make intuition check-ins a regular part of your routine, even for small decisions.
- **Check for Alignment:** Does your intuitive guidance align with your values, goals, and overall purpose? If not, it might be worth exploring further or seeking additional guidance.

Remember, your intuition is your inner compass, always guiding you towards what is best for you. By learning to tune in and listen to its wisdom, you can make more aligned decisions, overcome challenges with greater ease, and live a life that feels authentically yours.

Example: Career Change Decision

Let's say you're considering a career change, but you're unsure if it's the right move. You could do an Intuition Check-In by focusing on the question, "Is this career change aligned with my purpose?"

As you tune into your body, you might notice a sense of excitement in your chest and a feeling of lightness in your stomach. When you listen to your inner voice, you might hear whispers of encouragement or see images of yourself thriving in this new career. These could be signs that this change is indeed aligned with your purpose.

On the other hand, if you feel a sense of dread or heaviness in your gut, or if your inner voice expresses doubt or hesitation, that might be a sign to explore your options further or to reconsider your decision.

Trusting your intuition doesn't mean ignoring logic or practical considerations. It's about incorporating your inner wisdom into the decision-making process. By combining your intuitive guidance with rational thinking, you can make more informed, empowered, and ultimately fulfilling choices.

Day 30: Live with Intention

Congratulations, friend! You've made it to the final day of our 30-day journey. Take a moment to reflect on how far you've come. You've unearthed fears, released regrets, and discovered your purpose. You've practiced gratitude, cultivated self-compassion, and embraced imperfection. Now, it's time to bring it all together and truly *live* with intention.

What does it mean to live with intention? It's more than just setting goals or following a plan. It's about infusing every moment with purpose and meaning. It's about making conscious choices that align with your values, your dreams, and your authentic self. It's about waking up each day with a clear vision of what you want to create and taking deliberate steps to make it happen.

Living with intention doesn't mean that every day will be perfect or that you'll never face challenges. Life is full of unexpected twists and turns. But when you live with intention, you approach those challenges with a different mindset. You see them as opportunities for growth, not setbacks. You trust in your ability to navigate through them, armed with the tools and strategies you've developed over the past 30 days.

Imagine waking up each morning with a sense of clarity and purpose. Imagine feeling excited about your day, knowing that your actions are aligned with your values and goals. Imagine feeling confident in your decisions, trusting your intuition, and making choices that bring you closer to the life you desire. This is the power of living with intention.

In this chapter, we'll explore practical ways to integrate intentionality into your daily life. We'll discuss the importance of setting daily intentions, creating rituals that anchor you in the present moment, and making choices that move you closer to your dreams. We'll also delve into the power of mindfulness, gratitude, and self-compassion in supporting a life of intention.

By the end of this chapter, you'll have a clear understanding of how to live with intention, not just for the next 30 days, but for the rest of your life. You'll have the tools and strategies to create a life that is meaningful, fulfilling, and regret-free. So let's dive in and discover how to truly live with purpose, passion, and intentionality.

THE POWER OF INTENTION

Imagine your life as a ship sailing across the vast ocean of possibilities. Without a clear destination or a guiding compass, you're at the mercy of the winds and currents, drifting aimlessly and potentially ending up far from where you truly want to be. But what if you had the power to set your own course, to choose your destination, and to navigate your ship with unwavering focus?

That's precisely what setting intentions can do for your life.

Intentions are like the rudder of your ship, guiding your actions, decisions, and ultimately, your destiny. They are conscious choices about how you want to show up in the world, what you want to create, and who you want to become.

INTENTIONS AS A FOCUSING LENS

Think of your energy as a scattered beam of light. When you set an intention, it's like focusing that beam through a lens, concentrating its power onto a specific point. This concentrated energy can then be directed towards your goals, making them more likely to manifest.

For example, if your intention is to have a more productive day, you might focus your energy on specific tasks, minimize distractions, and create a structured schedule. By setting this intention, you're more likely to make choices throughout the day that support your goal, such as prioritizing important projects over busy work or resisting the urge to check social media.

INTENTIONS AS CONSCIOUS CHOICES

Living with intention means making conscious choices rather than reacting impulsively. It's about pausing before you act and asking yourself, "Does this choice align with my values and goals?"

Let's say your intention is to be more present in your

relationships. When your phone buzzes with a notification during a conversation with your partner, you pause and make a conscious choice to put your phone away and focus on the interaction at hand. This simple act of intention strengthens your connection with your partner and deepens your relationship.

INTENTIONS AS A SOURCE OF MEANING

Intentions are more than just a tool for productivity or goal achievement; they are a source of meaning and purpose. When we live with intention, we are actively participating in the creation of our own lives. We're not just passive observers; we're the authors of our own story.

Setting intentions that align with our values and passions can infuse our lives with a deeper sense of purpose. When our actions are guided by our intentions, we feel more fulfilled, engaged, and connected to our authentic selves.

PRACTICAL TIPS FOR SETTING INTENTIONS

Here are a few practical tips for setting powerful intentions:

- **Be specific:** Vague intentions lead to vague results. Instead of setting an intention to "be happier," be specific about what happiness looks like for you (e.g., "I intend to cultivate more joy in my life by spending time with loved ones and pursuing my creative passions").
- **Start small:** Don't try to change everything at once.

Begin by setting small, achievable intentions that you can easily incorporate into your daily life.
- **Write it down:** Writing down your intentions helps to solidify them in your mind and make them more real. Consider creating a daily intention journal or posting your intentions where you'll see them regularly.
- **Revisit and revise:** Your intentions are not set in stone. As you grow and evolve, your intentions may also change. It's okay to revisit and revise them as needed.
- **Be flexible:** Life is unpredictable. Don't get discouraged if you don't always live up to your intentions perfectly. The goal is to make progress, not to be perfect.

Remember, setting intentions is not a one-time event; it's a daily practice. Each morning, take a few moments to reflect on your values, goals, and priorities. Choose an intention that aligns with those aspects of your life and commit to living it out throughout the day.

By consciously choosing your intentions, you're taking control of the steering wheel of your life. You're no longer a passenger; you're the captain of your ship, charting a course towards a fulfilling, intentional, and regret-free life.

LIVING YOUR PURPOSE EVERY DAY

Now that you have a clear vision of your purpose, it's time to breathe life into it – to weave it into the very fabric of your everyday existence. Living your purpose isn't reserved for grand gestures or life-altering events; it's found in the small, intentional choices you make each day.

Think of your purpose as a guiding star, always there to illuminate your path, even on cloudy days. It's the thread that connects your actions, decisions, and interactions, infusing them with meaning and significance.

So how do you live your purpose every day? Let's explore some practical and accessible ways to bring your purpose to life:

1. Set Daily Intentions: Begin each morning by setting a clear intention for the day. This intention can be a simple phrase, a word, or even a feeling that aligns with your purpose. It could be something like "I will show compassion to others today," "I will pursue my passion project with focus," or "I will radiate joy and positivity." Write your intention down, say it out loud, or simply hold it in your heart as you move through your day.

2. Infuse Your Purpose into Your Routine: Look for ways to incorporate your purpose into your daily routine. If your purpose is to promote health and wellness, perhaps you start your day with a nourishing breakfast and a workout. If your purpose is to inspire creativity, maybe you spend a few minutes each day writing, painting, or playing music. If your purpose is to serve others, find small acts of kindness you can perform throughout the day.

3. Practice Gratitude: Gratitude is a powerful tool for living a purposeful life. When we focus on the good, we invite more abundance into our lives. Take a few minutes each day to express gratitude for the people, experiences, and opportunities that align with your purpose. This could be through journaling, meditation, prayer, or simply taking a moment to reflect on the blessings in your life.

4. Serve Others: Purpose is often found in service to others. Look for ways to contribute your unique gifts and talents to your community, your workplace, or the world at large. This could involve volunteering your time, mentoring someone, or simply offering a listening ear to a friend in need. Even small acts of kindness can make a big difference.

5. Pursue Your Passions: Remember those passions you identified earlier in our journey? Don't neglect them. Make time for the activities that bring you joy and ignite your soul. Whether it's painting, dancing, writing, gardening, or spending time in nature, engaging in your passions fuels your creativity and nourishes your spirit.

6. Embrace Challenges: Life isn't always smooth sailing, and challenges are inevitable. But when you live with purpose, you see challenges as opportunities for growth, not setbacks. Embrace them as a chance to learn, adapt, and become even stronger. Remember, the most meaningful growth often occurs outside our comfort zones.

7. Connect with Like-Minded People: Surround yourself with people who share your values and support your purpose. Join groups or communities that focus on the things you care about. Find mentors who can guide and inspire you. The company you keep can have a profound impact on your journey.

8. Celebrate Your Wins: Acknowledge and celebrate your achievements, no matter how small they may seem. Recognizing your progress reinforces positive behavior and keeps you motivated to continue pursuing your purpose. Share your wins with loved ones, treat yourself to something special, or simply take a moment to bask in the glow of your accomplishment.

9. Be Kind to Yourself: Remember, living with purpose doesn't mean being perfect. It's okay to have off days, to make mistakes, or to feel discouraged at times. Be kind to yourself, practice self-compassion, and remember that your journey is unique. There's no right or wrong way to live your purpose, as long as you're moving in the direction that feels true to you.

10. Reflect and Adjust: Take time regularly to reflect on your journey. Are your actions aligned with your purpose? Are you making progress towards your goals? Are you happy and fulfilled? If not, don't be afraid to adjust your course. Your purpose may evolve over time, and that's okay. The key is to stay connected to your inner compass and make choices that feel authentic and meaningful to you.

Remember, living with intention is a choice. It's a commitment to making the most of each day, to using your gifts and talents to make a difference, and to creating a life that you're proud of. It's a journey that takes time, effort, and dedication. But it's also a journey that is incredibly rewarding and fulfilling.

EXERCISE: DAILY INTENTION SETTING

Ready to supercharge your days with purpose and intention? This exercise is your secret weapon. It's a simple yet powerful practice that can transform how you approach each morning, each decision, and ultimately, your life.

WHAT IS A DAILY INTENTION?

Think of your daily intention as your North Star for the day. It's a guiding principle, a chosen attitude, or a specific quality you want to embody. It's not about adding another task to your to-do list; it's about setting the tone for how you want to *be* throughout the day.

WHY SET DAILY INTENTIONS?

1. **Focus and Clarity:** An intention acts as a filter for your thoughts and actions. It helps you stay focused on what truly matters, preventing you from getting sidetracked by distractions or negativity.
2. **Alignment with Purpose:** Your daily intention is a bridge between your big-picture purpose and your everyday actions. It helps you live your purpose, one day at a time.
3. **Mindful Living:** Setting an intention encourages you to be more present and aware throughout the day. You'll find yourself checking in with your intention, asking yourself, "Is this choice, this action, this thought, aligned with my intention?"
4. **Positive Mindset:** A well-crafted intention can uplift your mood and outlook. It sets a positive tone for the day, making you more likely to attract positive experiences.

HOW TO SET YOUR DAILY INTENTION

1. **Connect with Your Purpose:** Take a few moments to revisit your purpose statement. What is the overarching theme or goal that drives you?
2. **Choose a Word or Phrase:** Based on your purpose and what you want to cultivate in yourself, choose a word or short phrase that resonates with you. Some examples:
    - **Purpose:** "Make a difference."
    - **Passion:** "Embrace creativity."
    - **Growth:** "Learn something new."
    - **Connection:** "Cultivate meaningful relationships."
    - **Peace:** "Find calm amidst chaos."
3. **Make it Personal:** Your intention should be meaningful to you. Don't just choose a word because it sounds good; choose one that sparks a fire within you.
4. **Write it Down:** Take a pen and paper (or your favorite digital tool) and write down your intention. Keep it somewhere you'll see it throughout the day – your bathroom mirror, your desk, or your phone's wallpaper.
5. **Reflect and Reconnect:** Throughout the day, pause and check in with your intention. How is it showing up in your thoughts, actions, and interactions? Are you living in alignment with it?

Example:

Let's say your purpose is to inspire and empower others. Your daily intention could be:

- "Empower through kindness."
- "Lead with compassion."
- "Inspire through authenticity."

Now, as you go about your day, you'll be more mindful of opportunities to embody that intention. You might offer a listening ear to a friend in need, speak up for a cause you believe in, or simply share a smile with a stranger.

TIPS FOR EFFECTIVE INTENTION SETTING:

- **Keep it Simple:** A single word or short phrase is often more powerful than a lengthy statement.
- **Make it Positive:** Focus on what you want to cultivate, not what you want to avoid.
- **Start Your Day:** Set your intention first thing in the morning to set the tone for the day ahead.
- **Be Flexible:** If your intention doesn't resonate with you on a particular day, feel free to change it.
- **Reflect and Adapt:** At the end of the day, reflect on how well you lived up to your intention. Use this reflection to refine your practice for the next day.

YOUR DAILY INTENTION IS YOUR DAILY CHOICE

Remember, your daily intention is a choice – a choice to live a more purposeful, mindful, and fulfilling life. It's a choice to show up as your best self, even when faced with challenges. It's a choice to create a life that you won't regret.

So, choose wisely, my friend. The power to create your reality lies within you.

Conclusion

Congratulations! You've completed your 30-day journey toward mastering fear, following your purpose, and living a regret-free life. You've dug deep, faced your shadows, and emerged stronger, more confident, and more aligned with your authentic self. Give yourself a well-deserved pat on the back.

Remember those nagging doubts that kept you awake at night? The regrets that haunted your thoughts? The fear that held you back from taking action? They haven't disappeared entirely – and they may never. But they've lost their power over you. You've learned to recognize them, challenge them, and make choices that align with your values and goals.

You've created a powerful toolkit filled with daily practices that empower you to navigate life's challenges with grace and resilience. You've discovered your "why" and crafted a purpose statement that serves as your guiding light. You've learned to embrace your imperfections, celebrate your strengths, and cultivate a mindset of gratitude and self-compassion.

The journey hasn't always been easy. There may have been days when you stumbled, doubted yourself, or wanted to give up. But you persevered. You faced your fears, learned from your mistakes, and kept moving forward. And that, my friend, is the true essence of living a regret-free life.

YOUR JOURNEY BEYOND 30 DAYS

This 30-day guide is just the beginning. The tools and strategies you've learned are meant to be integrated into your daily life, not abandoned once the 30 days are over. Make these practices part of your routine, like brushing your teeth or eating breakfast.

Remember, living a purposeful life is an ongoing process. It's about continuously learning, growing, and evolving. It's about staying connected to your values, passions, and dreams. It's about making conscious choices that align with your authentic self.

EMBRACING A LIFELONG COMMITMENT

As you continue your journey, remember these key takeaways:

1. **Embrace Your Fears:** Fear is a natural part of the human experience. Don't let it paralyze you. Instead, use it as fuel to step outside your comfort zone and pursue your dreams.
2. **Let Go of Regret:** The past is the past. Forgive yourself for any mistakes you've made and use your experiences as lessons for growth.
3. **Discover Your Purpose:** Your purpose is your unique gift to the world. Take the time to discover what truly

lights you up and how you can use your talents to make a difference.
4. **Cultivate Self-Belief:** Believe in yourself and your ability to achieve great things. Silence your inner critic and replace negative self-talk with positive affirmations.
5. **Take Action:** Don't let fear or doubt hold you back. Take small, consistent steps towards your goals every single day.
6. **Build Supportive Relationships:** Surround yourself with people who uplift you, challenge you, and believe in your potential.
7. **Practice Gratitude:** Focus on the good in your life and express gratitude for your blessings.
8. **Embrace Change:** Life is constantly evolving. Be open to new experiences, opportunities, and perspectives.
9. **Never Stop Learning:** Invest in your personal and professional growth by continuously learning and expanding your knowledge.
10. **Live with Intention:** Make conscious choices that align with your values and purpose.

THE POWER OF "NO MORE WHAT IFS"

When you embrace a life of "no more what ifs," you unlock a world of possibilities. You gain the freedom to pursue your dreams, the courage to face your fears, and the resilience to overcome any obstacle. You become the author of your own story, creating a life that you'll look back on with pride and satisfaction.

Remember, this journey is not about perfection. It's about

progress, resilience, and the unwavering belief in your potential. It's about making choices you won't regret and living a life that is authentically yours.

So go ahead, my friend, and step boldly into your destiny. Embrace your purpose with everything you've got, chase those dreams like they're already yours, and make a decision right now to live a life free from the shackles of "what if." The world is waiting for you to rise up and shine—brighter than ever, unapologetically, and with all the fire God placed within you. This is your moment. Don't hold back.

CONNECT WITH ME:

- www.instagram.com/iamvonleshia

Milton Keynes UK
Ingram Content Group UK Ltd.
UKHW021459301024
450479UK00011B/242